— HIGHER —
EDUCATION

Published by Mindstir Media, LLC
45 Lafayette Rd | Suite 181| North Hampton, NH 03862 | USA
1.800.767.0531 | www.mindstirmedia.com

Printed in the United States of America
ISBN-13: 978-0-9988740-6-7
Library of Congress Control Number: 2017907111

— HIGHER — EDUCATION

The Stories Behind the Founding of the
University of Bridgeport
College of Chiropractic

written by Francis Zolli, D.C., Ed.D., D.Sc(H)

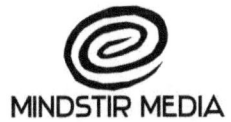

MINDSTIR MEDIA

DEDICATION

This book is dedicated to Ernest G. Napolitano and Neil Stern, the men who created the New York Chiropractic College. Their vision, courage and tenacity established the foundation upon which was built the University of Bridgeport College of Chiropractic.

ACKNOWLEDGEMENTS

I would like to acknowledge the contributions of the following individuals during the completion of this work:

Alana K. Callender

Rob Rop

Jillian Russo, Psy.D.

Paula Wiseman

Euie Ting Zambuto, Esq.

Adelia Zolli

Stephan J. Russo

INTRODUCTION

It has been over twenty five years since work was initiated on starting the first university affiliated chiropractic degree program in the United States. Since those original efforts began, circumstances have changed which have lead me now to write this book. Individuals originally associated with the project, either because of sickness or death, no longer play an active role in influencing the fortunes of either the chiropractic profession or the University of Bridgeport. Probably the greatest insight which has developed over the years has been my understanding of what really happened.

The foundation of this work is information found in my diary and original correspondence exchanged between principals, agencies and others. Diary entries reflect activities that occurred at the time. My comments are not supported by reference information. They are my opinions and interpretations of what was happening at the time. They are a snap shot of what happened, flavored by the emotion engendered by the activities at that time. The names of individuals in my diary, are published in this book as long as those individuals were in a public position, germane to the history of the project.

Diary entries are preceded by the date or dates covered in the entry and validated, where appropriate, by reference material. The narratives which follow diary entries are italicized and in parentheses. These statements reflect my recollection of events while such memories remain vivid in my mind, unencumbered by age or influenced by revisionist history. These thoughts are not supported by reference material.

For instance, one story I was told which has a direct bearing on the University of Bridgeport - College of Chiropractic has no supportive reference information. The story was told to me by a principal in the interaction. According to the press release issued in October 1989, the University Board of Trustees approved a planning process, which if successful, would culminate in the establishment of the first university based chiropractic program in the United States. An individual reading this press release might conclude the process leading to this announcement entailed many meetings of the administration, the accumulation of data from a variety of sources internal and external to the University, as well as consultation with representatives of the chiropractic profession about chiropractic education and the chiropractic profession.

What really happened went more like this.

The president of the University of Bridgeport was undergoing a chiropractic examination. During the examination, the doctor noted the muscles of the patient were extremely tense. The doctor questioned the cause of the tension and the president replied the University Board of Trustees had decided to close the nursing program and it was now the president's responsibility of replacing it with a new program in the health care field.

"Why don't you replace it with a chiropractic college," the doctor asked.

The president countered,"Where is the closest chiropractic program?"

"In Long Island, but it is moving to upstate New York," came the reply.

"No," the president persisted, "in Connecticut."

"There are no programs in Connecticut," the doctor explained. "The closest programs are located in New York, Illinois or Georgia."

"No programs in Connecticut?! No programs close?! We should look into this."

The doctor quickly responded, "If you'd like, I can introduce you to a local chiropractor who has experience with chiropractic education. He might be able to help you."

"I would appreciate it if you could arrange a meeting. Thank you."

And so it began. Well not really.

It really began …

TABLE OF CONTENTS

Transformation

Daniel David (D.D.) Palmer, the individual credited with founding chiropractic, started teaching healing methods in 1896[1], while practicing as a magnetic healer. Although the subject matter of his lessons might not have been chiropractic, his lecturess and practice would most certainly have been a type of healing which opposed traditional allopathic theory and practice. As a result he became a target of the medical establishment. Heinrich Matthey, M.D, a member of the Scott County Medical Society, would spend the next decade harassing both D.D. and his son, Bartlett Joshua (B.J.) Palmer. Matthey wanted to eliminate all drugless healing in Iowa, on the grounds such "irregular" practitioners constituted an unscientific and hazardous risk to the public welfare.[2]

Before there were laws which regulated the practice of chiropractic there were schools of chiropractic where students learned theory and practice. The dissonance between theory and practice was discovered by B.J. Palmer in 1903, when he was indicted for "publicly professing to cure and heal without having procured and filed a certificate of the Board of Medical Examiners." The indictment was focused on the practice of chiropractic and did not prevent the teaching of chiropractic![3] Afterwards, the diploma issued by the Palmer infirmary declared the holder was competent to Practice and Teach Chiropractic.[4] As students graduated from chiropractic programs, the number of schools increased. From Palmer's original school in 1896, the number of schools grew to 17 in 1906 and by 1924, 64.[5] Between 1895–1995, there were in excess of three hundred chiropractic degree programs in the United States and Canada.[6] Most of these schools lasted a limited time and benefited their owners more than the profession. Since the inception of chiropractic there has been a need to teach students the theory and practice of chiropractic. As students graduated they entered private practice and began to influence the laws which would define the practice of chiropractic. This influence, which occurred on a state and national level, was dependent upon the education the student received in chiropractic school and the type practice which resulted from that education. Those institutions led by visionary leaders withstood the test of time, met the internal and external challenges to the profession and those institutions which survived, continue to shape chiropractic education today.

The external challenges to the chiropractic profession throughout the 20th century were best identified in 1976 when five chiropractors, Chester Wilk, Michael Pedigo, Patricia Arthur, Steven Lumsden, and James Bryden brought a legal suit against the: American Medical Association (AMA), American Hospital Association (AHA), American College of Surgeons (ACS), American College of Physicians (ACP), Joint Commission on Accreditation of Hospitals (JCAH), American College of Radiology (ACR), American Academy of Orthopedic Surgeons (AAOS), American Osteopathic Association (AOA), American Academy of Physical Medicine and Rehabilitation (AAPMR), Illinois Medical Society (IMS), Chicago Medical Society (CMS), Medical Society of Cook County (MSCC), H. Doyl Taylor, Joseph A. Sabatier, M.D., H. Thomas Ballantine, M.D., and James H. Sammons, M.D., for violation of anti-trust law.(Wilk et al. vs. AMA et al., 1976).[7]

Among the specific offenses charged were refusal by the American Medical Association (AMA) and the other defendants ... to permit MDs and DOs to: refer patients to chiropractors, accept referrals from chiropractors, treat patients in cooperation with chiropractors, share office space, collaborate in research, teach at chiropractic colleges, lecture at their professional programs, and publish in chiropractic journals. The AMA also colluded to deny chiropractors hospital privileges and refused to take their radiographs. Efforts by the AMA were not limited to clinical interaction. They sought to persuade private insurance companies to deny coverage for chiropractic services, and exerted group pressure in an improper, illegal, and sham effort to obtain executive, administrative, judicial and legislative action by the federal and state governments adverse to the chiropractic profession.[8]

While these efforts came to light in 1976, the AMA initiated efforts to eliminate the chiropractic profession as a rival and threat to allopathic care in 1924. The actions of the AMA, though focused on the chiropractic profession, did not become organized until 1967 when the AMA Committee on Quackery established a plan to ensure the U.S. Office of Education did not recognize a chiropractic accrediting agency. This plan attempted to exploit the split in the chiropractic profession between straights and mixers.[9] The AMA realized the value of federal recognition of a chiropractic accrediting agency, as well as the threat of a unified chiropractic profession in terms of legislative efforts and health care policy.

The journey to accreditation by the chiropractic profession originally started in 1935 when the National Chiropractic Association (NCA) created a Committee on Education. Over time, this committee became the NCA Council on Education. This effort by the NCA was countered by the International Chiropractors Association (ICA) establishing the Chiropractic Educational Commission, which later became the Association of Chiropractic Colleges. It was the NCA Council on Education and the Association of Chiropractic Colleges which vied for federal recognition as the accrediting agency for the chiropractic profession.

Before federal recognition of the Council on Chiropractic Education (CCE), chiropractic colleges were approved by the profession's trade associations. While such approval made marketing material for the schools more impressive it also signaled the orientation of the school to chiropractors who were a source of student referrals. Trade association accreditation had no practical impact on chiropractic education. Professional association approval did not affect the finances of students. Chiropractic students were unable to secure federal loans or grants. As a result, chiropractic students had to work, while attending school, to pay their tuitions. The tuitions at chiropractic colleges remained low, enough to pay the expenses of the schools, but hardly enough to build the cash reserves necessary for growth.

The first significant milestone in the path to federal recognition of a chiropractic accrediting agency was the success of the National College of Chiropractic (NCC) in obtaining regional accreditation through registration with the state education department in New York.

"The New York Education Department has approved the professional education program of the National College of Chiropractic, Lombard, Illinois. This is the first chiropractic education program in the country to be approved by the Department under the requirements of the law which became effective January 1, 1968. As a result, persons completing the approved program will be eligible for admission to the New York professional licensing examination in chiropractic."[10]

Because of this milestone, NCC students who were residents of New York could qualify for federal loans and grants because the New York Education Department was recognized by the U.S. Office of Education, a division of the Department of Health, Education and Welfare, as a regional accrediting agency.[11]

The AMA was quick to respond. Ernest B. Howard, M.D., Executive Vice President of the AMA wrote: "… the American Medical Association… sincerely requests that the New York Board of Regents reconsider its approval of the profession education program of the National College of Chiropractic, Lombard, Illinois. We believe such approval is a disservice to the public in general, the health care consumers in particular and, above all, to the integrity of the accreditation system in the United States."[12]

The orientation of a chiropractic school was largely the standard by which the college gained trade association approval. A school aligned with the traditional teachings of the Palmers was termed straight. Straight schools were approved by the Association of Chiropractic Colleges. A school which mixed additional therapies with chiropractic was a mixer school and approved by the NCA. Both of these organizations had petitioned the federal government to be recognized as the chiropractic accrediting agency and both had been found lacking. The National College of Chiropractic which had achieved regional accreditation by the State of New York was approved by the National Chiropractic Association (NCA). By 1971 the NCA had become the American Chiropractic Association (ACA) and the ACA's Council on Education formally separated from the parent organization and became incorporated as the Council on Chiropractic Education (CCE), an autonomous body. The separation of the ACA Council on Education from the parent organization was accomplished to address a concern of the United States Office of Education (USOE). The federal government had been opposed to political organizations influencing an accrediting agency. The Association of Chiropractic Colleges had previously separated from the International Chiropractors Association, to ensure compliance with the USOE.

Despite the individual efforts of the Association of Chiropractic Colleges and the Council on Chiropractic Education to address the ongoing concerns of the USOE, neither could claim to represent the profession nationally. Both agencies approved five schools, half the programs in the nation, although the Association of Chiropractic Colleges (ACC) schools represented a larger percentage of total chiropractic students (72%) nationally. A series of meetings between the organizations occurred to discuss the possibilities of merger, "or methods, procedures and criteria to achieve a one voice representation for the chiropractic colleges."[13] Additional meetings were unable to satisfy the USOE's unwillingness to recognize two chiropractic accrediting agencies.

The ever-present AMA, requested and received approval to testify against the petitions of the CCE and ACC, reviewed the applications of both, and was granted 30 minutes of testimony before the USOE against each chiropractic agency.[14]

Commissioner T.H. Bell wrote in 1974, "I concur with the recommendation of the Committee and I am pleased to inform you that the Accrediting Commission of the Council on Chiropractic Education hereby is added to the Commissioner's list of Nationally Recognized Accrediting Agencies and Associations for one year."[15]

The struggle for federal recognition of a chiropractic accrediting agency is an example of the inability of chiropractic leaders to find common ground between the different points of view within the chiropractic profession. The split into straights and mixers is a schism which has plagued the profession since its inception. The controversy has influenced licensing legislation as chiropractors attained licensure throughout the country over a period of sixty years. It affected the lobbying efforts of chiropractic trade associations on the state and federal levels. It provided the AMA a focal point to advance its agenda to contain and eliminate the chiropractic profession.

The medical establishment and the chiropractic establishment created the circumstances which challenged the growth of chiropractic education in the twentieth century.

The Columbia Institute of Chiropractic (C.I.C.) was founded by Frank E. Dean M.B., D.C. in New York City in 1919. Dr. Dean was the chief administrator of the school until his death in 1958. The Columbia Institute of Chiropractic was the first non-proprietary school in the chiropractic profession.[16] Since chiropractic had no legal status in New York, the school's nonprofit charter was granted by the State of Delaware.[17] From 1919 until 1921 the Institute was housed on 72nd Street in Manhattan. In 1921 the Board of Trustees of Columbia purchased a four story building at 261 West 71st Street. This became the new home of the Columbia Institute of Chiropractic. A second building, 263 West 71st Street was purchased in 1923.[18]). These two modest facilities were the home of the Columbia Institute of Chiropractic for the next 40 years.

In 1954, the Columbia College of Chiropractic in Baltimore, Maryland, consolidated with the Columbia Institute of Chiropractic of New York City. The Columbia College was the first to initiate the two year pre-professional requirement.[19] The consolidation of the schools was part of NCA's plan to upgrade the quality of chiropractic education. Both institutions were small, but the Columbia Institute of Chiropractic had a larger student population and greater potential to draw future students being located in Manhattan. Both schools had been approved by the ICA's Chiropractic Education Commission.

The 1954 *Columbian*, the publication of the senior students of both programs, was dedicated to Frank E. Dean. On the dedication page, Dr. Dean was referred to as the program's director and the students' "Chiropractic Father." The students pictured in the book number 25. Seventeen were identified as residents of New York or New Jersey and six resided in Maryland or Pennsylvania. There were two African-American students pictured in the book, one male and one female. These students were listed as residents of Bermuda and the Republic of Panama.[20]

The co-dedication of the '54 *Columbian* was to Dr. Lorraine Welch. The dedication page refers to Dr. Welch as our own "Mabel," a reference to Mabel Palmer, B.J.'s wife, and a connection between Columbia Institute of Chiropractic and the Fountainhead, the Palmer School of Chiropractic (PSC).[21] The dedication page went on to praise Dr. Welch for traveling several times each week between both programs, without remuneration. Dr. Welch was the wife of Frank Dean. At the time of his death, she became the chief administrative officer of the Columbia Institute of Chiropractic.

The faculty pictured in the book were overwhelmingly chiropractors.

There was one PhD listed as a faculty member and possibly one M.D. While the PhD is listed as being assigned to the Department of Bacteriology, the faculty member listed as a doctor with no identifying credentials is assigned to the Department of Neurology. The professional anonymity of the doctor might have been necessitated by the hostile attitude of the AMA. Openly affiliating with chiropractors could cost an allopath professional relationships, and was a violation of the AMA Code of Ethics. The balance of the faculty were listed as being assigned to the Departments of: Anatomy, Special Anatomy, Physiology, Neurology, Chemistry, Roentgenology, Physical Diagnosis and Gynecology. The 1954 *Columbian* was the last jointly published by the Columbia College of Chiropractic and the Columbia Institute of Chiropractic.

Chiropractic education was changing, largely due to the efforts of John J. Nugent, the Education Director of the NCA. Dr. Nugent was a graduate of the Palmer School of Chiropractic, even though he had been expelled by B.J. Palmer because of "discourtesy to the President."[22] He was, however, reinstated by the faculty. His basic contribution to the chiropractic profession were the educational standards he authored and implemented throughout the profession. It was John J. Nugent, along with another NCA official, Dr. Emmett Murphy, who established contact with the United States Office on Education, which would eventually lead to recognition of the Council on Chiropractic Education.[23]

The 1955 *Columbian* was published by the senior class of the Columbia Institute of Chiropractic. The number and demographics of the faculty remained the same as the previous *Columbian*, with one exception. The faculty member who had attained a PhD was no longer listed in the book. There are 11 graduates pictured and the chiropractic faculty taught the majority of the courses in the curriculum, including all the basic sciences. The Columbia Institute of Chiropractic maintained approval by the Education Commission of the International Chiropractors Association (ICA) and would stay politically aligned with the traditional element of the chiropractic profession throughout the struggle for federal recognition of a chiropractic accrediting agency.[24]

On November 29, 1959, Ernest G. Napolitano was appointed by the Board of Trustees to the position of president, replacing Lorrain Welch.

Ernest G. Napolitano (EGN) was a 1942 graduate of the Palmer School of Chiropractic.[25] Dr. Napolitano, or Nappy, as he was known to both friends and enemies, like most PSC alumni was influenced by his relationship with B.J. Palmer. He was, however, a master politician. He had been president of the Atlantic States Chiropractic Institute.[26] At this point in his professional life he maintained loyalty to the straight orientation by which he had been trained and practiced, yet he maintained his independence of opinion.

The appointment of Dr. Napolitano was followed by the renovation of the school's existing buildings, which was completed in 1961.[27]

As part of Nugent's plan to upgrade the quality of and strengthen chiropractic education mergers between schools were arranged. Financially weaker schools were absorbed by schools which were financially stable. The Atlantic States Chiropractic Institute (ASCI) merged with the Columbia Institute of Chiropractic in 1964. As it had done ten years previously with the Columbia College of Chiropractic, the Columbia Institute of Chiropractic had absorbed a financially weaker program, thus strengthening chiropractic education in general. Both ASCI and C.I.C. had been approved by the ICA's Education Commission.[28] Another merger proposition between the Columbia Institute of Chiropractic and the Chiropractic Institute of New York (CINY) did not succeed. After a series of meetings and the dissemination of information to the chiropractic profession, talks were broken off when Columbia refused to accept CINY's demand for equal representation on the Board of Trustees.[29] The Chiropractic Institute of New York eventually merged with the National College of Chiropractic and the Columbia Institute of Chiropractic continued to function and grow in New York.

The C.I.C. *bulletin 1962–64*, indicated the school had been approved by the Education Commission of The International Chiropractor's Association and the American Association of Chiropractic Schools and Colleges. Faculty were not listed and tuition was listed as $214 per term for day students and $240 per term for evening students.[30]

Enrollment in the Columbia Institute of Chiropractic primarily consisted of local students from the five boroughs of New York and the state of New Jersey. The cost of tuition multiplied by the modest number of students matriculating in C.I.C. provided enough revenue to sustain the school, but no base upon which the school could grow. The focus of training at C.I.C. was changing. In 1964 Dr. Napolitano resigned from the ICA's Board of Control and announced his school would seek accreditation from the Council on Education of the newly formed American Chiropractic Association.[31] The accreditation focus would be a radical departure from previous efforts expended by Columbia and it's affiliates, the Columbia College of Chiropractic (CCC) and the Atlantic States Chiropractic Institute (ASCI). Dr. Napolitano, the master politician, did however maintain membership in the Association of Chiropractic Colleges. When the struggle for federal recognition was raging, the secretary-treasurer of the ACC was Ernest G. Napolitano. When the ACC and CCE had their meetings to discuss merger, the ACC representative was Ernest G. Napolitano. The Columbia Institute of Chiropractic was the smallest program accredited by the ACC.[32]

Despite the change in orientation, the Columbia Institute of Chiropractic still faced challenges in achieving academic legitimacy. The physical plant of the school was small and remained in New York City. The number of students in the school remained small. The faculty had grown to include 59 members. All save one were doctors of chiropractic. Dr. Napolitano understood the need to diversify the faculty. He also understood the sentiment of the chiropractic faculty and profession at large, to start hiring PhD's would dilute the focus of chiropractic education.

After Dr. Napolitano assumed the presidency, Dr. Welch, remained at C.I.C. as an educational consultant, and was warmly regarded as Columbia's First lady. The administration of the school maintained personnel from the institutions which had merged with Columbia over the years. As a result there was definite resistance on the part of Columbia personnel and faculty to the direction Ernest G. Napolitano was taking the school. Despite the new direction upon which C.I.C. was headed, the program remained small. In addition to the 11 graduates pictured in the 1968 *Columbian* there were an additional 31 students pictured.[33]

To accommodate the anticipated expansion of the student body, in 1973 the Board of Trustees directed the administration to enter into a contractual agreement with the New York Institute of Technology

(NYIT) of New York City and Old Westbury. Effective with the entering class of January 1974 the academic program of the Columbia Institute of Chiropractic would be conducted on the campus of NYIT in Long Island, New York. This contract changed the face of the Columbia Institute of Chiropractic faculty forevermore.

Now the instruction of chiropractic students in the basic sciences were PhD's. While this may have ensured students were receiving a better caliber education, the chiropractic faculty who previously taught these courses were sure the subject matter was not taught in alignment to the principles of chiropractic. Just as they feared and had been predicted by chiropractors all over the country, chiropractic education was being watered down. The basic science faculty were not interested in chiropractic at all. They believed their jobs were teaching the subject matter that was their expertise. Applying this information to the practice of chiropractic was the responsibility of the students learning the material.

Despite the grumbling and resistance of the faculty, Dr. Napolitano knew the agreement between the schools afforded C.I.C. a foundation upon which to grow. The Columbia Institute of Chiropractic now had a contractual relationship with an institution of higher learning having status with the Board of Regents of the State of New York, as well as regional accreditation by the Middle States Association of Schools and Colleges. Neither of which status was enjoyed, at that time, by a chiropractic program.

The Columbia Institute of Chiropractic was making progress in addressing the academic standards of the Commission on Education of the Council on Chiropractic Education. These standards addressed: Objectives, Organization, Administration, Scholastic Regulations, Curriculum, Faculty, Clinical Experience, Library Program, Instructional Aids and Equipment, Research, Physical Facilities, Laboratories, Research, Postgraduate and Related Professional Education and Ethical Practices. The United States Office of Education had recommended the CCE require of its accredited schools to list in their college catalogues not only the degrees held by the faculty, but also the year and institution which had awarded each degree. The *bulletins* of the Columbia Institute of Chiropractic, starting in 1974, identified all faculty consistent with this recommendation.[34]

The faculty at this time (1974) included: Frank De Giacomo, D.C., C.I.C. '65, Philip Striano, D.C., C.I.C. '67, and Peter Giacalone, D.C., C.I.C., '64. Each of these individuals would play pivotal roles in the evolution of the Columbia Institute of Chiropractic. James McDonnell, D.C., C.I.C., '56 had been a member of the administration of the college for years. He had been eclipsed as Dean of the College by Neil Stern, D.C., C.I.C., '68. The interpersonal relationships each of these individuals maintained with Dr. Napolitano, are an indication of the autocratic style in which Dr. Napolitano controlled the fortunes of the Columbia Institute of Chiropractic.

Dr. Napolitano shared with Arnold Cianciulli, D.C., and myself the story behind Dr. McDonnell's demotion and exile. It seemed Nappy had a cousin who had matriculated at C.I.C. and he was not the strongest student academically. At the end of the fall term the student was academically separated from the school by the dean, Dr. McDonnell. Dr. Napolitano was not notified of the action that had been taken. As a result, when Dr. Napolitano went to Christmas Eve dinner at the home of the student who had just been academically dismissed from the program, he received a frigid reception. Upon inquiring as to the why the family was so upset, he was told what had transpired. The next morning, Dr. McDonnell was no longer the Dean of the Columbia Institute of Chiropractic. Dr. McDonnell's transgression occurred at the end of the fall semester of 1970. His name as a member of the institute's administration disappeared and did not reappear in a bulletin until 1980. By this time, the Columbia Institute of Chiropractic had become the New York Chiropractic College.

In 1980, Dr. McDonnell resumed his position as dean of the college. Some faculty resented the manner in which Dr. McDonnell was removed. They felt Dr. Napolitano overstepped his authority and penalized Dr. McDonnell simply for doing his job. Dr. Napolitano's perspective on this situation was that Dr. McDonnell was not fired, as he should have been, and stayed on the payroll. It was Nappy's school and he had not been shown the proper respect. His action was similar to that taken by B.J. Palmer when he dismissed John Nugent for his discourtesy to the president of Palmer.

By the time Jim McDonnell was re-appointed dean, Neil Stern had risen to the position of Executive Vice President of the College. After his graduation from C.I.C., Dr. Stern joined the administration as the associate director of adjusting service.[35] Dr. Stern's next position in the administration was Dean and Director of Adjusting Service.[36] By this time, Dr. McDonnell had committed his indiscretion and was not even listed in the College bulletin as a member of the administration.Dr. Stern was then appointed as Dean and Clinic Director, Dr. McDonnell was still not listed.[37] Dr. Stern then became Dean and Chief of Clinical Staff.[38] When Neil Stern was appointed Executive Vice President, Dr. McDonnell was re-appointed Dean.[39] During this process of passing seasoned faculty while accruing more responsibility and authority over the faculty, Dr. Stern was seen as Nappy's "boy." Whenever Dr. Napolitano wanted anything accomplished, and accomplished thoroughly and correctly, he would assign the task to Dr. Stern and it was done. Despite the accomplishments achieved by the school, all because of his work, Dr. Stern could not get the respect of the faculty.

Although numerous individuals were listed as members of the administration of the Columbia Institute of Chiropractic when the school prepared for CCE accreditation, the actual administration of the institution was:

President–Ernest G. Napolitano, D.C.
Dean & Clinic Director–Neil Stern, D.C., F.A.C.C.

They were on campus every Monday, Wednesday, and Friday. Both practiced on Tuesday, Thursday, and Saturday. When they were on campus, Dr. Napolitano's Cadillac would be parked in a reserved space just outside the entrance to the Graham House, the college's administration building, and Dr. Stern's Corvette would be parked across the parking lot from Nappy's. On days Dr. Napolitano was not on campus no one parked in his spot, it was reserved for the president of the college. Once the president of the student government parked his car, an orange Corvette, in Dr. Napolitano's spot. It was a Tuesday and he knew Nappy would not be on campus. Unfortunately, not five minutes after he parked his car, Dr. Napolitano's Cadillac pulled up to the administration building. Nappy pulled his car behind the orange Corvette parked in his reserved space, ensuring the vehicle could not move, exited his car and entered the building, going directly to his office. He exited campus about six hours later, finally releasing the offending vehicle, and its disrespectful owner, from their captivity.

Each day they were on campus would start with both Dr. Napolitano and Dr. Stern meeting in Nappy's office for at least two hours. The contents of the meeting would range from topics such as purchasing real estate for the school, to state and national chiropractic politics to securing professional accreditation, to achieving an absolute charter, to dealing with the mundane issues of running a college. Every detail of the process was reviewed and a timetable for completion was developed. Dr. Stern then made the plan work, to the satisfaction of Dr. Napolitano. While Neil Stern made sure the t's were crossed and i's dotted, it was Dr. Napolitano who arranged the circumstances, applied the political pressure, made the connections and attended the meetings that allowed the results to be realized.

Evidence of Dr. Napolitano's reliance on Dr. Stern can be discerned from a memo sent to the staff of the Columbia Institute of Chiropractic dated July 27, 1977. The purpose of the memo was to advise the recipients of the reprinting of the college bulletin and their individual assignments. Dr. Stern was assigned 13 individual sections of responsibility, in addition to editing the entire document. The submissions of the individual sections were to be made to the office of the president, but the final editing responsibility would be Dr. Stern's.[40]

Another memo, dated February 26, 1985, reports the results of an inspection Dr. Napolitano made on the occasion of his visit to the Levittown clinic. The second paragraph of the memo emphatically states Dr. Stern had been personally authorized by Dr. Napolitano to correct all the deficiencies noted in the report. Naturally, the other recipients of the memo were expected to aid in the process. More specifically, each individual receiving a copy of the memo was to follow Dr. Stern's orders to ensure the clinic was clean.[41]

The balance of the administration consisted of Mollie Donovan, her sister Edith Mazzie, and Alice Armstrong. Each of these women were intensely loyal to Nappy and would report any campus event to him that occurred on a day he was not on campus. When the Executive Committee was created as a standing committee of the college, Mollie Donovan was a member, eventually being listed as vice-chair of the committee. The clinic receipts were submitted daily to Mollie and her sister, Edith. The directors of the clinical facilities who made the receipt submissions would take the opportunity to provide the ladies with an update on the latest news from the clinics. This news was transmitted to Dr. Napolitano, who always seemed to know what was happening all over campus.

The second reason for Nappy's apparent omniscience was Alice Armstrong. Anyone wishing to meet with Dr. Napolitano had to make an appointment with Alice. Naturally, Alice would need to know the reason for the request, and queried the individual. Usually the person was only too happy to provide the details as to why Dr. Napolitano was being sought to intervene in the matter. Appointments were never granted on the day they were requested. This enabled Nappy to find out the root of the problem, and obtain various opinions on how the situation would impact the institution. By the time the meeting occurred, the visitor was amazed at how thoroughly Nappy had analyzed the situation and how comprehensively his response solved the dilemma.

Once the move to Long Island had been accomplished, additional real estate was purchased to support the anticipated growth of the academic program. The Greenvale clinic was opened in 1976, followed by the Levittown clinic two years later. With the clinical training of students being accomplished on Long Island, there was no longer any need to maintain the Manhattan clinic, and in September 1978, the Manhattan facility was sold, severing the ties of the Columbia Institute of Chiropractic with the past. The sale of the Manhattan property was predicted by faculty to have an adverse effect on the clinical skills of the students in the program. Interns would never see the variety or number of patients they could have in Manhattan. Both Long Island clinics eventually developed substantial patient rosters to provide students the clinical experience they required.

My personal relationship with Dr. Napolitano started in February

1977. My mentor, Arnold Cianciulli, D.C., had introduced legislation in New Jersey. At the committee hearing on the proposed legislation, C.I.C. students testified against the bill. Arnold was furious and asked that I write a report to the administration of C.I.C. about what was happening in the student body. The controversy over a straight or mixer orientation to the school raged daily on campus. Students maintained their own opinions, and were influenced and supported by members of the faculty as well as speakers at outside seminars. I wrote the report and delivered it to the administration, with a copy to Dr. Cianciulli. After several days I was summoned to a meeting with Dr. Napolitano and Dr. Stern. At that meeting Dr. Napolitano read to me the letter he wrote in response to my report—all seven pages.[42] Naturally the letter, though addressed to me, was written for Dr. Cianciulli, but since I wrote the report, I had the privilege of listening to the response. Dr. Napolitano's response was a methodical, systematic dissection of each point I had made in my emotional report to Dr. Cianciulli. The thorough, meticulous manner in which Dr. Napolitano responded was an indication of how seriously he considered and reacted to any criticism against his school, even criticism levelled by a second-semester student.

It was the first time I had ever been in his presence. To arrive at his desk one had to walk passed an informal area adorned with a leather couch and chairs. There was a large globe in that area, which when opened, presented a fully stocked bar. (I did not find out about the bar for several years.) Between the furniture and Dr. Napolitano's desk was a conference table with eight wooden chairs. After traversing the length of the office, a visitor sat at the desk of Ernest G. Napolitano. There was a bay window behind his desk and a door next to the bookcase against the wall. All the windows in the room were covered with drapes. A plush rug covered the floor. The room was impressive and designed to intimidate any visitor, who understood upon entering the room that the occupant was an individual of gravitas. If your visit was one wherein good news was to be conveyed, walking up to the desk was easy. If the visitor had done something to incur the wrath of Dr. Napolitano, the walk could be interminable. During the course of our relationship, I experienced both. When Dr. Napolitano read the rebuttal to my report we sat at the conference table.

Several weeks later, I had the opportunity to meet Dr. Napolitano again in his office. The candidates for student government were invited to meet with Dr. Napolitano, and I was running for vice president. He looked at me with faint recognition, and before he could say anything I told him we had previously met. He nodded and walked to the next candidate.

Dr. Napolitano had distinctive stationery and a distinctive autograph. Both the stationery and autograph were reminiscent of B.J. Palmer. He was also an eloquent speaker and an excellent writer. The circumstance dictated the type of stationery used. The letter-sized stationery was ecru and simply said at the top, under the logo and address of the institution—Office of the President. Short memos were typed on beige stationery, which had Dr. Ernest G. Napolitano emblazoned at the top. Nappy was a stickler for protocol. Any act of kindness to himself or the college was always acknowledged with a thank-you note. If a member of the staff achieved a level of recognition outside the college, they would receive a congratulatory letter. As president of the student council, I received three letters from Nappy, one thanking me for running a successful Unity Day, and two others thanking me for helping to make our accreditation process successful.[43]

As president of the student body, it was my responsibility to arrange student escorts for members of the CCE site team. In addition, I was given the privilege of reading the self-study and attending planning meetings related to the site visit. It was at these meetings I started working with the members of the faculty and administration.

The Columbia Institute of Chiropractic was granted Recognized Candidate for Accreditation (RCA) status in 1978 by the Commission on Accreditation (COA) of the Council on Chiropractic Education (CCE). As a result of this achievement the school was issued a provisional charter by the Regents of the University of the State of New York resulting in the institution being renamed the New York Chiropractic College (NYCC). NYCC was securing, on its own, what NYIT had originally brought to the institution.

In January 1979, the New York Chiropractic College was granted accredited status by the Council on Chiropractic Education and in October was granted an absolute charter from the Regents of the University of the State of New York.[44] The real success of professional accreditation was enabling the New York Chiropractic College to be eligible for Bundy Aid. This was a program which provided direct, unrestricted financial aid to independent post-secondary institutions in New York State. The annual entitlement provided to each school was based upon the number of degrees conferred by the school in the previous year. The original award rate was $2400 for each doctoral degree conferred by the program.[45]

I started working as a clinician at NYCC in January 1980. In a short six months I was promoted to Director of the Levittown Clinic. In my letter of appointment, Dr. Napolitano indicated I had a full charge position at the facility. In the same letter, the position of Clinic Chief of Staff had been discontinued.[46] I assumed the responsibilities of the position held by Libero Violini, CINY '51, and enabled the clinic to function more efficiently. This position also strategically placed me in a position where I could interact with Nappy's personal representatives on a regular basis. Each day I would bring the clinic receipts to the Graham House and engage in a conversation with Mollie and Edith. I normally started the interaction by asking, "Is he in a good mood?" Edith thought my irreverence was funny and we engaged in light banter about campus personalities and situations. My comments were usually colorful and comedic, causing the ladies to try to stifle their laughter. Their office was next to Nappy's and there was always a chance he would walk in. On the several occasions he did interrupt our conversations. Mollie, Edith and I immediately became very serious, and after he exited the room, we carried on like children whose parents had just disciplined us. The irreverent banter started our relationship and was the foundation upon which the relationship grew.

My advancement to Clinic Director was not embraced by the senior members of the faculty. Jim McDonnell felt I was a Nappy puppet, just like Neil Stern, placed on the faculty as a political favor to Arnold Cianciulli. Frank De Giacomo and Peter Giacalone believed I was too young to be given the responsibility of running the clinic. The fact that Frank Langilotti, D.C., CINY '57, an "old-timer" on staff had been the chief of staff,[47] did not help my standing with the old guard. Phil Striano, who practiced in New Jersey, agreed with the sentiments of his colleagues, but in all fairness thought I should be given a chance succeed or fail based on my own efforts. Fortunately, stationed in the Levittown clinic, my inter-action with the on-campus faculty was minimal, but they were watching.

Despite all the progress that had been made under Ernest G. Napol-itano, the faculty maintained a smoldering resentment to the way the college was run. Nappy and Neil were on campus three days a week—the three days chiropractic faculty practiced. As a result, faculty could never meet with the administration to discuss any topic unless they took time out of their practice. Faculty felt they had limited influence on policies and procedures implemented at the college. Everything was discussed, planned and implemented by Dr. Napolitano and Dr. Stern. Dr. McDon-nell, who was senior to Dr. Stern in terms of service to the school, was not consulted on any issues, a fact he bitterly resented.

After years of planning, meetings with architects and the Old Brookville zoning board, and securing professional accreditation and an absolute charter, the college held ceremonies opening the newly con-structed academic center in September 1980. The 40,000 square foot structure contained four large classrooms separated by collapsible walls. When these walls were collapsed, the result was an auditorium which could hold up to 600 people. In addition the facility contained two chi-ropractic technique labs, an x-ray learning lab, faculty and administra-tive offices and a student lounge/cafeteria.[48] An additional wing to the academic center constructed to house a human anatomy laboratory was completed in December 1981.[49]

The resistance and resentment of the faculty never changed. Fac-ulty members consistently complained about the manner in which the administration ran the school. Despite the advances achieved by the administration, the faculty never seemed to be satisfied. Among the issues of contention were: class schedules were not transmitted to faculty with enough notice for faculty to make the arrangements necessary to sustain their private practices. There was no job security. Faculty could be replaced with a phone call from the administration, without any explana-tion other than the faculty member's service was no longer needed. This dissatisfaction reached its peak in January 1983.

The administration called a mandatory faculty meeting on a Sunday prior to the start of the January term. The reason for a Sunday meeting was to ensure maximum attendance by the chiropractic faculty, most of whom practiced around their faculty schedules. Maximum attendance by the faculty meant the topics discussed would be disseminated to the faculty, providing the faculty the opportunity to communicate their ideas directly to Dr. Napolitano. From the administration's point of view, maximum attendance, by the chiropractors on staff would ensure the information transmitted would not be misinterpreted. All chiropractic faculty were asked to sign an attendance roster, which was collected by Dr. Stern. There was no such requirement imposed on the basic science faculty.

Dr. Napolitano took the stage and eloquently described how NYCC students were the beneficiaries of their basic science classes being taught by a cadre of well-credentialed, dedicated faculty. He went on to explain that this faculty were a large part of the success in NYCC being accredited by the CCE. Furthermore, he hoped this relationship would continue and as a result, the college would grow and prosper and become the finest chiropractic program in the world.

The members of the chiropractic faculty in the audience waited for an acknowledgement of their contribution to the college. It never came.

After the meeting, the chiropractors in attendance noted the complete lack of respect afforded the chiropractors. They also noted the number of basic science faculty in attendance was minimal, even though the substance of Dr. Napolitano's remarks were directed toward them. It was known the compensation paid to the basic science people was much higher than the pay offered the chiropractic faculty. This was the final insult. After years of enduring Dr. Napolitano's high-handed, autocratic ways, low compensation and disrespect, the chiropractic faculty had had enough. A committee of faculty would be formed to investigate compensation rates at the other chiropractic schools and develop a position paper to be presented to Dr. Napolitano. The presentation of the position paper would start the process of rectifying the complaints of the faculty. Since such a committee would be considered treason at NYCC, the principals involved had to act swiftly and secretly.

The first matter of business would be to select representatives. Recognizing the transition occurring in the faculty Frank De Giacomo, C.I.C. '65, and Frank Langilotti, CINY '57, were elected to represent the perspective of the older members. Paul Cadolino, NYCC '79, and Frank Zolli, NYCC '79, represented the points of view of the younger members of the faculty.

The committee met numerous times to discuss the various issues that required reconciliation. Data was collected from other institutions. It never occurred to the members of the committee, that presidents from other schools might share this information with Nappy.

As a result of these meetings a document was developed which addressed the issues. It was presented to the faculty at a meeting held at the Levittown clinic. The document consisted of eight pages and contained the signatures of twenty six members of the chiropractic faculty. The various pages of the document addressed the issues of concern, most importantly salary and contracts. At that time, it was agreed upon by all in attendance (everyone who signed the petition) that the document would be delivered to Dr. Napolitano on the day before he was to leave for the CCE meeting. This day was picked to force Dr. Napolitano to the table. He would be forced to the table because he would not want the embarrassment of a strike known by the public and chiropractic profession. Dr. Napolitano was also the president of the CCE at this time.[50] It was agreed by all faculty at the meeting that if anyone participating in this action was fired, everyone else would strike.

The information was delivered to Alice Armstrong on Thursday February 12, 1983.

As anticipated, Dr. Napolitano was enraged. He immediately tried to break up the ringleaders. He called Frank Langilotti, who was traveling on a lecture tour and unavailable. Paul Cadolino was not yet in his office and missed Nappy's call.. Dr. Napolitano called the Levittown clinic and spoke with Andy Lacerenza, D.C., the clinician on duty, who he verbally abused, and threatened to fire all of us. Andy called me in my Jersey City office to advise me of what was happening. I then called Frank De Giacomo and told him Nappy was enraged and attempting to fire us all. Dr. Napolitano was committed to ending this insurrection quickly. He called Bob Matrisciano, the president of the New York State Chiropractic

Association (NYSCA) and a member of the Board of Trustees to enlist his help in replacing the members of the faculty who signed the petition and threatened to strike.

While this process was occurring, Nappy received a call from Frank De Giacomo, who later shared the contents of the call with me. Frank had joined the faculty in the sixties and was well respected by students and faculty alike. The two spoke about their relationship and the changes occurring in chiropractic and the world, at which time, Nappy asked a question.

"Frank, if I asked you a question, would you give me a truthful answer?"

"Of course, Ernest, (Frank had the privilege of calling Nappy by his first name), what's the question?"

"Who is responsible for this petition?"

"Do you truly want to know?"

"I do," said Dr. Napolitano.

Dr. De Giacomo responded, "You are."

Dr. Napolitano then offered Dr. De Giacomo a special deal to call off the revolt. DeGiacomo refused and the call was terminated.

All day long phone calls were made and received by members of the faculty, some from Dr. Napolitano and some from other faculty members. Four weeks into the semester and Dr. Napolitano was prepared to replace a significant percentage of the faculty because they challenged his authority. Communication was constant and the threat of the strike held.

At approximately 4:00 pm, I called Dr. Napolitano, who accepted my call.

I attempted to start the call with civility by asking, "How are you, sir?"

"Not well," was the response.

"Could I help in clarifying the issue?"

He then went on tell me how he had treated me like a son and I had betrayed him.

"You know something, Zolli? You're a bum."

"That may be true, sir, but I think it would be more productive if we stay focused on the current situation."

"I have been focused on the current situation all day."

"Well, now that we're talking about it, perhaps I can help you."

"I'll let you know when and if I ever need your help."

"I'm here if you need me." He hung up.

At 5:00 pm I received a call from Dr. Napolitano himself advising me that he would meet with the faculty committee after he returned from the CCE meeting. I thanked him for his decision and stated I looked forward to the meeting. I then started the phone chain to tell the faculty what had transpired.

At the CCE meeting Dr. Napolitano met with Dr. Cianciulli and advised him I was a traitor. Arnold's relationship with Nappy had dated back to a time when the state of New Jersey was going to revoke its approval of C.I.C. graduates to practice in the Garden State. After which time, they became close friends and confidents. Arnold advised Nappy that he was wrong. If I had taken such a strong position against him, it was in the best interest of the college. Dr. Napolitano did not like hearing this, but because Dr. Cianciulli was on the ACA Board of Governors and the New Jersey Board of Medical Examiners, Nappy did not want to lose him as an ally. As a result, I was not fired, but Nappy did make my life miserable.

The largest issue on the table was compensation. In 1983 the federal minimum wage rate was $3.35/hour.[51] Starting salary for D.C. faculty was $6.00/hr. Starting salary for basic science faculty was $40.00/hr. The general sentiment of the chiropractic faculty was a willingness to work for low wages because this was their contribution to the profession. In addition, all were practicing and receiving revenue from their practices.

A review of the document shows the obvious deference to which Dr. Napolitano was treated. The front page of the document, signed by the representatives of the faculty, stated the respectful suggestion of the representatives that the proposed schedule was to be used at the discretion of the president.[52]

Page two of the document states it is not the intention of the chiropractic faculty to dictate the pay scale for the entire NYCC community. The document went on to state, in the second paragraph, that should an exceptional faculty member be recruited by NYCC, it is the prerogative of the president to "make the arrangements necessary to secure the services of the new faculty member," The new faculty member would be compensated reasonably with the standards being applied to NYCC faculty. Such a provision was interpreted by Dr. Napolitano as an infringement of his authority as president of the institution.

The basic guidelines outlined in the document called for an increase in base salary from $6.00/hour to a minimum of $12.00/hour. Diplomates and authors would also be compensated at a different, higher rate. While 12.00/hour was higher than the prevailing pay scale, and lower than the 40.00/hr paid to the basic science faculty, it reflected the attitude of the faculty.

The balance of the document consisted of an outline of items to be included in the contracts to be awarded faculty. The contract start date was to be April 1983. At that time NYCC was on a trimester teaching schedule. Included in the contract would be the responsibilities of the faculty member, a review schedule of faculty performance. Faculty would be paid on the basis of hours worked, and would need to maintain office hours without compensation.

The faculty member would be advised four weeks before the start of the semester what his or her schedule would be. If the college altered the teaching schedule of a faculty member, the incumbent would need to be offered the position before it was assigned to a new faculty member. The faculty member would be evaluated at least twice per year by students and whomever the college administration designated.

A position of faculty dean was created to be appointed by the president based on a list of nominees submitted by the faculty. One responsibility of the faculty dean would be to assist the academic dean in developing the class semester schedule.

The meeting with Dr. Napolitano started icily. The older faculty representatives were effusive in their gratitude of being able to meet. Dr. Napolitano responded by expressing his disappointment at the turn of events which led to the current situation. He then began addressing the specifics of the document. The faculty representatives were immediately uncomfortable and unwilling to engage in the discussion. As a result, the meeting was a matter of Dr. Napolitano dissecting the document. There was not a line in the proposal he found acceptable. The salary rates would need to be reviewed in light of their impact on the budget. The salary increases to be allocated to diplomates and authors was eliminated out-right as being too self-serving since only Frank De Giacomo and Frank Langilotti had published books at this time. Nappy also took this occasion to inform the representatives that he was aware of the meeting held to ratify the proposal where the faculty response was not unanimous. In addition to the lack of unanimity, the number of faculty signing the proposal was not a majority of the faculty, therefore the provisions in the proposal to be included in contracts to be offered faculty could not possibly become a reality. Nappy was letting us know he had an informer on the faculty, and while we had prevailed in securing this meeting, any future efforts would be fraught with unpleasant consequences. At this point the meeting was approaching adjournment when Dr. Napolitano, looking directly at Drs. De Giacomo and Langilotti, again expressed hurt as a result of our collective actions. He then looked at Paul Cadolino and stated, "You're too young to understand these things." In his own way, Nappy absolved Dr. Cadolino of any wrongdoing. He never looked at me at all during the meeting.

Nappy knew that although the faculty had maintained solidarity for one day, they would not band together to fight him again. All he needed to do was appear reasonable and willing to compromise, and that would satisfy the majority of the faculty. Now all he had to do was claim to be working on the situation, and start the process of eliminating, in his mind, the ringleader of the revolt.

Because of the threatened strike base salaries were raised. The other elements of the proposal were soon forgotten by the faculty and never realized. Dr. Napolitano's retribution, however, was quick and efficient. One visible move which taught faculty the penalty for crossing Dr. Napolitano was my removal as Director of the Levittown clinic. This action was taken after it became apparent I was not doing my job. My inefficiency at doing my job resulted from my inability to respond to directives or submit reports requested by personnel in the Graham House, none of which I had ever received. This allowed Nappy the opportunity to compile a file which justified his action. It also allowed him to have evidence that his action was based upon objective decision making, not vindictiveness. I was persona non grata in the Graham House. In that I had no reason to deliver receipts to Mollie and Edith, I was discouraged from visiting their office. Prior to my being marooned, Mollie Donavan told me that despite what had happened, "He really likes you." Dr. Napolitano did not wish to speak with me so I had no reason to speak with Alice Armstrong. Other staff who worked in the administration building would be unwilling to be seen talking with me.

In the clinic I was not assigned my own office, but given a desk in the director's office—where I could be watched and monitored. My status as a pariah dragged on for months. Finally, I submitted my resignation to Dr. Napolitano.

One afternoon, after I had submitted my resignation, I received a call in the clinic.

"Let's talk. I received your letter. Bring all your baggage." That was the entire conversation. Naturally, I recognized the voice and immediately drove to Dr. Napolitano's office. It was approximately 5:30 pm, so all staff were gone for the night. For the next five hours I listened to Ernest G. Napolitano. We went to dinner at a local restaurant. He told me tales of B.J. Palmer, Vinton and Hugh Logan, William Werner, securing licensure in New York, and the future of NYCC and the chiropractic profession. At the end of the talk, he asked, "Do you still want to resign?"

"No, sir."

"That's good because I have no intention of accepting your resignation." At which point he tore my resignation letter into pieces.

From that point on, Dr. Napolitano and I were friends. We never spoke of my indiscretion of leading a faculty revolt. He was a guest at my wedding and visited my home for dinner, where I was privileged to hear stories of chiropractic history. At one "history" lesson Nappy mentioned Palmer School of Chiropractic was once racially segregated. He went home, afterwards and attempted to find the catalogue that would validate his statement. When he was unable to locate the necessary documentation he contacted Russell Gibbons, a chiropractic historian, who confirmed Dr. Napolitano's statement, in writing. Nappy was a stickler for detail.[53]

The New York Chiropractic College was accepted as a candidate for accreditation by the Commission of Higher Education of the Middle

States Association of Schools and Colleges in 1983. Accredited status was granted in March 1985.[54]

My reclamation from the pariah heap did not occur overnight. When my replacement as Clinic Director suffered a heart attack and had to step down from the position, I resumed the responsibilities of the office, without being officially re-appointed. This gave me access to Mollie, Edith and Alice once again, and as a result, Nappy. The journey back ended on October 1, 1984, when I was appointed Chairman of the Clinical Science Division of the College. This position had been announced at a staff meeting several weeks earlier. At that time, I privately asked Dr. Napolitano if he would have any objections to my applying. He liked that I had shown the appropriate respect by asking his opinion before I took action. My appointment letter for the position was inaccurate, containing a mistake. As a result, a second accurate letter was sent, with an explanation of why the first letter needed to be corrected.[55]

While my duties were focused on the clinical sciences, my position gave me direct access to Dr. Napolitano. As a result, assignments were directed to my attention where Nappy wanted constant access to the progress being made in addressing the issue. While this appointment cemented my return to Nappy's good graces, it also raised the apprehensions of senior faculty and administration.

A month after my appointment as Division Chair, Dr. Napolitano appointed me as Chair of the Chiropractic Science Review Committee. Members of the committee included Neil Stern, James McDonnell, Frank De Giacomo and Philip Striano. The significance of my appointment as chair was not lost on the committee members. The competition that had long festered between Dr. McDonnell and Dr. Stern now included me.

One day, after meeting with Dr. Stern, I was walking through the Graham House when I came across an executive chair. The first floor of the Graham House was largely reserved for the president. When a visitor entered the building, the visitor was greeted by a receptionist. There were two chairs across from the receptionist's desk in which the visitor could wait. The second floor contained Dr. Stern's office and the offices of his staff, as well as other administrators. One large office was occupied by his administrative assistant and the other was occupied by two additional secretaries. A visitor entering the building for a meeting with Dr. Stern was usually sent to the office of his administrative secretary, after she had been alerted by phone of the visitor's presence.

After my meeting had ended I proceeded to his administrative assistant's office to schedule another meeting. In her office was a desk she used when collating reports and documents. At the desk was an executive chair. The leather was nicked slightly on the right hand, but aside from this one blemish, the chair looked impressive. I inquired as to who owned the chair. It belonged Dr. Napolitano. I sent him a memo requesting to use the chair. "To say the least, I am honored that you decided to use my chair—use it in good health, dear friend," was the response.[56] I proudly exhibited the chair to anyone and everyone who visited my office, always noting the original owner. That chair remained my chair throughout my time at NYCC.

Another time I dismissed an adjunct faculty member whose attendance on campus to teach her classes was compromised by her inappropriate priorities of sleeping and addressing personal problems. The faculty member called Neil Stern to complain about what had transpired. I was called in to the office of the executive vice president and told I could not fire people. When I voiced disagreement, Dr. Stern picked up the phone, said he was sorry to have to do this and called Dr. Napolitano to report what I had done. "Zolli knows what he is doing," was the response from Dr. Napolitano and I never had any additional issues with Dr. Stern. The adjunct faculty member who had been terminated was replaced by a new adjunct faculty member, Anthony Onorato, D.C.

If a prospective faculty member was seeking employment, they would frequently contact Dr. Napolitano directly. I would receive a note which read in part, "It (the applicant's CV) is not being sent to you for the purpose of encouraging employment." If employment was to be encouraged, the communication would occur in person, between myself and either Dr. Napolitano or Dr. Stern. There was never a paper trail.

When a member of the core science faculty was accused of plagiarism, Dr. Napolitano requested I investigate the matter and report the results of my investigation to him. Dr. Napolitano, after reviewing the results of my investigation concurred that the similarity between the documents reviewed was not coincidental. The faculty member met with Dr. Napolitano, then resigned.

My prominence as a member of the administration continued to grow, as did the resentment of the other, older members of the administration and faculty.

At the beginning of the 1985 spring term, Bud Passero, a prominent Connecticut chiropractor and close personal friend of Dr. Napolitano, was invited to lecture at NYCC. Dr. McDonnell was assigned the responsibility of introducing the speaker, an assignment he resented. He was not shy about letting Dr. Passero know that he had better things to do and that if people wanted to invite speakers to campus, they should be available on campus when the speakers arrive. This information made its way to Nappy who determined such disrespect needed to be immediately addressed.

I was summoned to Dr. Napolitano's office the next morning where Dr. McDonnell, Dr. Stern and I were treated to a vintage Napolitano tirade about never airing our dirty laundry in public. My presence at the meeting was not well received by Dr. McDonnell.

By 1985 the New York Chiropractic College had risen to a position of prominence in academic circles. It had achieved professional accreditation, an absolute charter from the state of New York and regional accreditation. In February of that year, Dr. Napolitano retired from private practice. The day before he announced his retirement I made the following entry in my diary, "… Had a good meeting with Dr. Napolitano and … I hope Dr. Napolitano's message came through—he was never better; there is a certain sadness about the man now, but he is still Dr. Napolitano—his strength is quiet but firm; and all there; he is a good teacher in the best way, by example and I hope someday to be as good as he." Nappy remained energized by the constant flow of information that came his way from his personal sources, and as a result kept the staff very busy.

At the time, I did not realize Dr. Napolitano was teaching me how to run a college. I found out years later after I was admitted to the doctoral program in educational leadership at the University of Bridgeport. I sat through classes and read books on topics I knew from practical experience. From Nappy I learned how to conduct business, from school I learned the theories of why business should be conducted in this manner.

My diary entry for June 2, 1985: "Ernest G. Napolitano passed away." I had been called at home by Neil Stern and immediately drove to the Graham House. There, in Nappy's office, were Neil Stern, Jim McDonnell and Frank De Giacomo. Frank told me he had been offered the presidency of the college by the Board of Trustees (who were scheduled to meet this day), but turned it down. He said he advised Neil to do the same thing. Neil was attempting to get in touch with Mr. Hendrickson, the college's attorney. The main reason to contact Hendrickson was to find out if Dr. Napolitano had left documents or directives regarding a successor.

Dr. Stern was the Executive Vice President, so it was assumed he would take over. He was not well-liked by the faculty, through no fault of his own, he was seen as Nappy's hatchet man. He was not well-liked by other administrators who saw him as Nappy's boy. These individuals could not compete with Neil's abilities or his relationship with Dr. Napolitano. Some people, mostly faculty or administrative friends, thought Jim McDonnell should be the next president, because of his length of service to the school. Dr. McDonnell, however, had his own detractors on the faculty and within the administration. He was, by nature, a very negative person. For him, the question was not, is the glass half full, but how much poison is in the glass.

Drs. Stern, McDonnell and DeGiacomo had gone through Nappy's office looking for evidence of who Dr. Napolitano had designated as his successor. They had completed their search, without success, before I arrived at the Graham House. After a little time passed Drs. McDonnell and Degiacomo left to go home. Dr. Stern and I waited for attorney Hendrikson who had been summoned from the golf course.

Dr. Napolitano's will addressed the distribution of his estate without mentioning his preference for a successor. This was problematic. Allegedly Dr. Napolitano had indicated to some people Neil Stern would be his successor, while to others it would be Jim McDonnell, and to others, Bob Matrisciano would be the next president. None of these allegations could be proved. Nappy was great at telling different people different things about the same situation. In this way individuals believed they had gained Nappy's confidence and maintained a vital secret important to NYCC.

Dr. Napolitano also had great success making "secret" deals with people that were confidential and could be shared with no one. Afterwards, when the details of these deals became common knowledge, it became apparent to everyone that Nappy had maneuvered individuals to keep them at odds with each other by having them think their deal was more advantageous than that of their counterpart. Ernest G. Napolitano was a master politician, equally adept at handling members of the ICA or ACA, the CCE or the Board of Regents. He had the ability to keep people off balance, and as a result he maintained control of many situations simultaneously. Unfortunately, he was no longer around.

CONFLICT

There were two distinct challenges facing the administration of the New York Chiropractic College created by the death of Ernest G. Napolitano. The first was running the college. For the first time in over 25 years, the individual most responsible for the growth and development of the college was absent. The leader and visionary of chiropractic education in the northeast was no longer Ernest G. Napolitano. Administration and faculty who had been taking orders from Nappy for years, and resented each directive, now had to follow their own instincts on what to do and Nappy could not be blamed for their actions. Individuals who freely criticized Dr. Napolitano for his inaccessibility and secrecy, now became aware of the challenges of juggling multiple issues simultaneously.

The second, more problematic issue, was an apparent violation of CCE Standards concerning some members of the Board of Trustees. Previously, the Board of Trustees had been described as "… outstanding citizens who are donating their services to the chiropractic profession." This statement was the official position of the school, found in the Columbia Institute of Chiropractic *Bulletin 1962–64*.[1]

Dr. Napolitano had the intellect, vision and political savvy to transform the Columbia Institute of Chiropractic, but he needed something more practical to energize the process—money. The responsibilities of the board were described in the Columbia Institute of Chiropractic *Bulletin 1965–68* which stated, "… [The Board] establishes policies for the institution, passes on all structural changes or improvements and disbursements, and approves recommendations for changes in the Administrative and Faculty staff."[2] The Plan of Organization further states it is the responsibility of the president to, "maintain direct and continued communication with the Interim Committee of the Board of Trustees. This committee is composed of the Chairman and Vice Chairman of the Board."[3] The Columbia Institute of Chiropractic was controlled by the President and Chairman of the Board. Prior to this organizational plan being published and articulated by the institution, the President and Chairman of the Board of Trustees were one and the same person, Ernest G. Napolitano.[4]

The composition of the board changed over time. As membership on the board changed the roles of the board and administration became better defined. However the board was irrevocably altered with the addition of three C.I.C. faculty members, Robert Matrisciano, D.C., Gordon Heuser, D.C., and Rolla Pennell, D.C. Bob Matrisciano once confided in me that, in addition to advising Nappy on any number of issues, he was also a source of money whenever Nappy needed it for the school. He indicated the other Trustees who joined the board with him served in similar capacities.

Bob Matrisciano was a successful chiropractor practicing in Queens, New York. In addition to serving on the faculty of the Columbia Institute of Chiropractic, he became involved in chiropractic politics in New York State. As a result of his personal resources and his friendship with Ernest G. Napolitano, he was able to win the presidency of the New York State Chiropractic Association (NYSCA). In his capacity as president he was able to have pro-chiropractic legislation passed which directly benefited the school. Of particular importance was the legislation which allowed chiropractic students to use human cadavers in the study of anatomy. On the basis of this law being passed, there was no legal reason to stand in the way of the construction of anatomical facilities for the New York Chiropractic College.

Gordon Heuser and Rolla Pennell were business partners in a number of successful enterprises. The most prominent of their businesses was a practice management company named Clinic Masters. In addition, these doctors were also partners in Practice Masters and Doctor's Financial Fund.[5] Each of these business enterprises was successful and had chiropractic clients from across the country. Dr. Napolitano frequently spoke at seminars sponsored by these companies, and as a result, could advertise the accomplishments of the school to an audience which would otherwise be unaware of the New York Chiropractic College. Since chiropractors were a source of referrals for the school, these efforts by Dr. Napolitano were a way to possibly diversify the student population to include students from outside the New York-New Jersey - Connecticut area. The names of these Trustees were originally published in the 1975–76 *Bulletin* of the Columbia Institute of Chiropractic.[6] The statement regarding the

Trustees donating their services to the chiropractic profession is omitted in this publication.

Toward the end of his life, Dr. Napolitano realized he was losing control of the board of trustees to Drs. Heuser and Pennell. Two doctors had been added to the board. Mahlon Blake, D.C., and William Rousch, D.C. who were also clients of Clinic Masters. In addition, Dr. Pennell recommended his cousin, Winfield Salisbury to the board for membership. In his confidential and personal letter to Dr. Napolitano, Dr. Pennell identified his relationship with Dr. Salisbury, and stated the nominee would be "absolutely dependable in every way." He went on, "I believe he would make an ideal addition to our board and would be 100% loyal to you and your programs."[7] The official nominating letter to the search committee mentioned Dr. Salisbury's education and scientific background as his qualifications for board membership.[8] At the time of his death, Dr. Napolitano had agreed to endorse Roger Calton, the Clinic Masters' attorney for the next open board seat. As a result, this potential block of six votes could influence college policy, and could be even more formidable, if it combined with the interests of other trustees.

The first challenge confronting the administration of NYCC was the funeral and burial of Dr. Napolitano. Neil Stern busied himself making sure all the arrangements were perfect. In addition to notifying the various organizations to which Nappy maintained membership, other presidents of schools and political leaders on a state and national level were contacted. Arrangements were made with the funeral home, and the script for the funeral and following procession were developed. Dr. Stern also arranged to have Glen Cove Road and the Long Island Expressway (LIE), major roads in Long Island, closed for the funeral procession. As all these arrangements were being made camps were forming within the Board of Trustees regarding the selection of the next president. Within the college administration, Drs. McDonnell and DeGiacomo were poised to carve up the college, so that whoever became president, their experience and position would make them indispensable.

The first day of the wake shocked attendees because Dr. Napolitano's coffin was closed. The room was filled with flowers and mourners and rumors. The most prominent rumor was that Dr. Matrisciano would be named the next president. He was the current president of NYSCA. If he were to assume the presidency of the New York Chiropractic College, the combination of the two organizations under his control could pose a formidable political alliance to aid in the growth of the chiropractic profession in New York State.

After two days of viewing, the funeral was a standing-room-only event. Dr. Stern was able to arrange a police motorcade to accompany the funeral procession along the route to the cemetery. The repast was held on campus and Dr. Stern invited those in attendance to tour the place "Ernie had built." The funeral was attended by chiropractic dignitaries from across the country. Presidents from other schools were honorary pall bearers. There were officers of the American Chiropractic Association, International Chiropractors Association, the Council on Chiropractic Education and the chiropractic Associations in New York, New Jersey and Connecticut. Anyone in attendance who toured the facilities could not help but be impressed by the spacious rooms supported by modern technology. Anyone who had trained in Manhattan at the two brownstones that were the Columbia Institute of Chiropractic, or at the Chiropractic Institute of New York, which had merged into the National College of Chiropractic, or the Atlantic States Chiropractic Institute which had become part of C.I.C. had to realize chiropractic education, in the form of the New York Chiropractic College, had traveled light years from the modest facilities of their training._

Ernest G. Napolitano always seemed to be the target of criticism of many people at NYCC and in the chiropractic profession. His actions were certainly criticized by the faculty and administration at NYCC. While not directly criticizing Dr. Napolitano, the American Medical Association constructed obstacles which made his life more challenging. Theodore Roosevelt, who never knew Nappy, encapsulated his focus, energy and achievements in the face of the adversity he faced when the president wrote:

"It is not the critic who counts, not the man who points out how the strong man stumbles, or where the doer of deeds could have done them better. The credit belongs to the man who is actually in the arena, whose face is marred by dust and sweat and blood; who strives valiantly; who errs; who comes short again and again, because there is no effort without error and shortcoming; but who does actually strive to do the deed; who knows great enthusiasms, the great devotions; who spends himself in a worthy cause; who at the best knows in the end the triumph of high achievement, and who, at the worst, if he fails, at least fails greatly, so that his place shall never be with those cold and timid souls who know neither victory or defeat."[9]

Ernest G. Napolitano had to overcome the effects of the prejudice and ignorance of the AMA and its influence on legislation and educators. He had to overcome the ignorance and pettiness of chiropractors who opposed his vision simply because it was not theirs. He had to stabilize an educational program that subsisted on modest tuition and small enrollment. He supervised the renovation of the Manhattan campus when funds were a challenge. He supervised the move of the school to Long Island when it became obvious more space was required. He entered into a contractual agreement with the New York Institute of Technology which afforded the Columbia Institute of Chiropractic access to a world inaccessible to chiropractic education at the time. He supervised the procurement and building of a modern campus. Along the way, the New York Chiropractic College achieved professional accreditation from the Commission on Accreditation of the Council on Chiropractic Education. The college secured regional accreditation from the Middle States Association of Schools and Colleges. The New York Chiropractic College also secured an absolute charter from the Board of Regents of the State University of New York.

The day ended with Neil Stern and me having a drink at his yacht club, sharing stories of Nappy and discussing the future.

After five days of no classes out of respect for Dr. Napolitano, Monday started with a meeting between Frank DeGiacomo, Frank Langilotti, Jim McDonnell and myself. The three of my colleagues agreed they should support Jim McDonnell for president, even though they all agreed Neil would be easier to manipulate. I remained non-committal on the topic.

Dr. Langilotti informed us he had had lunch with Genevieve Klein (a Trustee who was strongly opposed to Dr. Stern's candidacy) and she advised him that selecting the president would be a long process. It was decided an Advisory Council would be formed to aid Dr. Stern in running the college. The purpose of this committee would be to ensure the stability and integrity of the institution, while the college endured the trials, tribulations and uncertainty of the presidential search process. The purpose of the Advisory Council was to benefit the college, and not the individuals on the committee.

The following afternoon, at a meeting of the Advisory Council, it was decided and agreed upon that everyone would support Dr. Stern for the presidency. Additionally, Dr. DeGiacomo would be named chair of the Division of Chiropractic, removing that responsibility from myself, and Dr. Langilotti would be placed in charge of postgraduate and continuing education. This arrangement was to install Drs. DeGiacomo and Langilotti, neither of whom liked Neil, in positions of authority. Their preference for president was Jim McDonnell, who wanted the job for himself. Assuming the presidency would be vindication for Dr. McDonnell, having endured years of disrespect by Dr. Napolitano.

The all-for-one mentality of the administration lasted for about a week. Jim McDonnell announced at a staff meeting he would be applying for the presidency. His rationale for his decision was if there were two internal candidates, it would increase the chances of one of them being selected. The other would then remain in his current position. This announcement met with the approval of Drs. DeGiacomo and Langilotti, both of whom who could understand and support Dr. McDonnell's reasoning.

The posturing of individual members of the administration as it related to the presidential search is an indication of their naiveté. For years, they had heard Dr. Napolitano tell them how he acted to influence the Board of Trustees. They made the mistake of confusing their abilities and stature with that of Dr. Napolitano's. While the Board of Trustees could be influenced by Nappy, they were not going to be influenced by Drs. Stern, McDonnell, DeGiacomo, or Langilotti. In addition, the unknown factor which could influence the selection of the president was the individual agendas of board members who would be making the ultimate decision. The functioning of the college was so insulated that the possibility of an external candidate emerging who might be elected president was never seriously considered by the senior members of the administration.

Dr. Stern raised the salaries of the members of the administration who had assumed more responsibility during the transition. He advised me, in lieu of additional compensation, to reduce the amount of time I spent at school. It became apparent that without Dr. Napolitano's presence, the senior members of the administration would be aligned against me, and Dr. Stern would act in any manner that ensured their support.

The first order of business, external to the college, was attending the annual CCE meeting. I accompanied Dr. Stern based upon his invitation. Drs. Heuser and Pennell, representing the board of trustees, were also along for the trip. This was the first experience Drs. Heuser, Pennell or myself had with the CCE. Dr. McDonnell had wanted to make the trip to start familiarizing himself with personalities associated with the CCE, making his presidential candidacy potentially more palatable to the Trustees. After hearing reports for years about interactions with the Council on Chiropractic Education and the Commission on Accreditation, as well as meetings with state and national trade associations, the members of the Board of Trustees knew Dr. McDonnell lacked the experience to interact with any off-campus organizations.

Dr. Heuser indicated the search for the next president had already begun, but in the interim the board had total confidence in Dr. Stern. There was no real substance to NYCC's appearance before the Commission on Accreditation at this time. The meeting had been scheduled months in advance, and was a mutual courtesy call. The members of the Commission expressed their sympathy on the loss of Dr. Napolitano to Dr. Stern, for dissemination to the entire NYCC community. On the other hand, the representatives of NYCC assured the Commission NYCC would be prepared for the next meeting in six months. It was understood that business as usual would prevail the next time we met.

I was asked by the editor of the *American Chiropractor* magazine to write a feature article on Dr. Napolitano. While researching my topic, I contacted Dr. Matrisciano for some anecdotes about Nappy. He provided many, all of them about the humanity of Ernest G. Napolitano. He spoke of Nappy the doctor, the clinician, the friend, the mentor. While it was Nappy's stature as an educator, politician, and giant in the field which got his picture on the cover of the magazine, the memories shared by those who knew and loved him were of the man. This article was the first time Bob Matrisciano and I ever worked together. It started a collaboration and friendship which would last for the next 30 years.

Frank Langillotti and I did not get along personally. This relationship began when I was a student. One day I was in an office for an appointment with the doctor who shared the room with Dr. Langilotti. Upon entering the room Dr. Langilotti reprimanded me for my lack of manners. When I attempted to explain why I was there, he flew into a rage, citing my disrespect as his reason for vacating the room.

When the doctor with whom I was supposed to meet entered the room, after having met Dr. Langilotti on the stairs, he asked me what had transpired between Dr. langilotti and myself. After I told him what had happened, he recommended I seek out Dr. Langilotti and apologize to him. The doctor also remarked Dr. Langilotti has a long memory and in matters he perceived as disrespect, could be very vindictive. I then went and apologized. From that point on, our interactions were strained but courteous.

Once I became a member of the faculty I became more aware of his administrative skill set.

I considered him to have great ambitions for himself and very limited abilities. I remember describing his administrative skills to the clinic staff once as an accident waiting to happen. As a result, I tried to minimize my interactions with him. Frank had served in a variety of administrative capacities during his career at NYCC, including Clinic Director, Dean of Continuing Education, and Clinic Chief of Staff, always being relieved of his duties because of one or more consistent miscalculations on his part. His latest quest was to again be re-appointed chief of staff of the clinics. In an effort to gain my support, which he knew he did not have and had little chance of receiving, .he approached fellow CINY alumnus Arnold Cianciulli. He shared the rationale that there should be a unified front of all individuals in the administration during this potentially turbulent time. Arnold, who did not have to deal with Frank on a regular basis, agreed with the logic and ordered me to make peace with Dr. Langilotti. This meant I should not be critical of Dr. Langilotti's performance, ideas, or actions going forward. My reticence to speak or criticize Dr. Langilotti did not extend to the other members of the administration.

In spring 1986, Dr. Frank DeGiacomo, the Director of the Chiropractic Division of the College wrote a memo to Dr. Langilotti, questioning the content of the clinic examination. Dr. DeGiacomo was questioning the lack of questions on the examination relating to chiropractic analysis or technique.[10] This inquiry started a cascade of responses by Drs. Langilotti and myself.[11] By now the Trustees' conflict had already boiled over and members of the administration spent most days on campus and in courtrooms. Nights were spent in Dr. Stern's office reviewing the day's accusations and facts, and planning our next moves. These meetings usually ended in the early hours of the morning. In these meetings an attack on a member of the administration by another administrator raised suspicions about the loyalty of the individual initiating the conflict.

The balance of 1985 was spent focusing on daily business, posturing by Advisory Council members and preparing for the next CCE meeting. An additional responsibility for administrators was added in regard to daily business. A budget process was created to ensure the Board of Trustees would be able to approve the operating budget for the next fiscal year. Previously, all financial matters presented to the Board of Trustees were confidential and limited to interaction between the board and the president. A November 18, 1985, letter to the Board of Trustees outlined the budget process which had been developed by Dr. Stern. In addition to citing the steep learning curve required by all members of the administration, Dr. Stern also noted, "To the best of my knowledge the Trustees had never been provided a 'proposed' budget, but were only given a 'year-end' report."[12]

At approximately the same time, in correspondence with J. William Nystrom, the Chairman of the Board of Trustees, Dr. Stern revealed the contract between NYCC and the New York Institute of Technology was scheduled to expire on August 31, 1989. As a result it was necessary to initiate actions which would make "NYCC a free-standing institution of higher and professional education."[13]

While preparing for the CCE accreditation hearing, information became available to the members of the Advisory Council that potentially jeopardized the accreditation of the institution. Based upon the documents and correspondence in the files, it became apparent members of the Board of Trustees were profiting, or attempting to profit, from the operations of the school based upon their position as Trustees. It was also apparent that Dr. Napolitano was complicit in these maneuvers.

After six months of preparation, the next meeting with the Council on Chiropractic Education arrived. Six months was not enough time to prepare the representatives of the college for what they heard. After years of achievement, growth and progress, the determination handed down was a shock. On January 28, 1986, the Commission on Accreditation of the Council on Chiropractic Education placed the New York Chiropractic College on confidential probation. In a letter to Acting President Stern, dated January 29, 1986,[14] Patrick H. Sullivan, Jr., D.C., the Chairman of the Commission on Accreditation identified the Trustees who appeared to be in violation of the Standards as:

Gordon Heuser, D.C.
Mahlon Blake, D.C.
Rolla Pennell, D.C.
William Rousch, D.C.
Harold Zerdin
Roger Calton

In a follow-up letter from Dr. Sullivan to Mr. Vito Forte, Chairman of the NYCC Board of Trustees, dated February 21, 1986, Dr. Sullivan states, "I am somewhat astonished at what seems to be surprise by members of your Board concerning longstanding Standards concerns the Commission has had with the New York Chiropractic College."[15]

Dr. Sullivan goes on to say these concerns were expressed in the June 1982 resolution of the Commission which was sent to "your College President and the Chairman of the Board."[16] Whatever information was transmitted to the President was kept secret. Whatever information was transmitted to the Chairman of the Board, it appears, never reached him.

Even before the actions of the Commission on Accreditation, it had become apparent to members of the college administration that Standards violations were being perpetrated at NYCC. Correspondence between

Dr. Napolitano and several Trustees, identified as confidential, gave the appearance of being unethical.[17] Student lists were confidentially sent to board members to help them solicit business.[18] Instead of action being taken by the board to resolve the concerns, evidence was mounting that the president was conspiring with the Trustees to maintain the status quo. Finally, the Commission had taken an adverse action against the college after having longstanding concerns go unheeded. The fact the college was in violation of the Standards was problematic. The fact this violation was a longstanding concern was devastating.

The inexperience of the Board of Trustees, without the firm hand and experience of Ernest G. Napolitano to navigate them through turbulent waters, then became woefully apparent. Based upon Dr. Sullivan's letters to Acting President Stern and Chairman Forte, Dr. Napolitano had been aware of the concerns of the Commission. In addition to not transmitting the Commission concerns to the Board of Trustees, he also never shared with anyone how he planned to resolve the situations.

At the next scheduled board meeting conducted on March 1, 1986, the six Trustees cited by the CCE were removed from the board. The action taken was based upon the advice of an attorney, skilled in pro-chiropractic litigation but ignorant of the bylaws of the college and Board of Trustees. The action taken was not on the board meeting agenda which had been transmitted to the membership in advance of the meeting. The Trustees removed had not been formally notified of the proposed action to be taken against them. As a result, these six individuals brought suit against the college, claiming they had been deprived of due process. Dr. Napolitano, in a potentially catastrophic situation, would not have acted in haste. The matter would have been legally researched and rehearsed by all the principals involved before any action was taken. The action taken would have been consistent with the processes required by law and reviewed and rehearsed to ensure everyone knew their roles in the proposed drama. Dr. Napolitano was not available to orchestrate the removal nor could he advise the board membership on how to take advantage of the established rules of the CCE. The Council on Chiropractic Education had an appeals process which the New York Chiropractic College could have used to buy time in an effort to resolve this conflict. Unfortunately, because of the inexperience of the Trustees with educational processes and procedures, and no one to guide them, their solution to the problem, though well-intentioned, only created chaos.

As a result of this action to remove board members, six Trustees who would have voted on the next president were no longer in office to vote. The future of the college was now listlessly floating on the seas of judicial indifference. The tsunami to follow would involve the courts, the state legislature, the Board of Regents, the students, faculty and administration of NYCC, the public and chiropractic media, and the chiropractic profession in New York State and the nation. The plot would unfold over a course of several months, and in the end, the band-aid applied as a solution would solve this embarrassment, and be the cause of the next one.

The Council on Chiropractic Education, based upon their academic standards, had identified six Trustees who were the cause of the concerns. Although it could not be proven in a court of law, the Clinic Masters block of the NYCC Board of Trustees controlled six votes. Five were directly affiliated with the Clinic Masters organization, Drs. Heuser, Pennell, Blake, Rousch, and their attorney, Roger Calton. In addition, Harold Zerdin, though not directly connected with Clinic Masters, was of a similar mindset as it related to making money from his position as a trustee.

In addition, Winfield Salisbury had been elected to the board based upon the nomination of Rolla Pennell. Dr. Salisbury's position on the Board was expected to be "100% loyal" to Dr. Napolitano and his programs.[19] Another Trustee who was sympathetic to the composition of the Board of Trustees because of his personal business interests was Louis Wein. Eight solid votes to select the president and establish policy for the institution were in the hands of the Clinic Masters block. This was the interpretation of the board composition which motivated the chairman and three other members to act.

To counter the Clinic Masters block of votes were four Italian-American Trustees: Robert Matrisciano, George Bonetti, Salvatore Abruzzo and the Chairman of the Board, Vito Forte. With the thought of accreditation revocation being a real possibility because of the longstanding concerns of the CCE, and the slim chance of the existing membership of the

Board of Trustees voting to correct the concerns, a decision was made by the four and members of the administration to create a situation where either the courts, or the Board of Regents, would become involved and protect the students of the New York Chiropractic College. To that end, informational meetings were held with faculty and students to explain to them the nature of the charges against the college.

The courts became involved immediately after the meeting of March 1, with suits and counter suits filed by Trustees against other Trustees. During the course of court hearings information was divulged which intensified the situation. An article appeared in *Newsday*, the local newspaper, on April 23, which announced the confidential probation status which had been imposed by the CCE to the students and public.

On April 24, Judge Stuart Ain ordered the re-instatement of the six trustees removed from the board. On the basis of the court overturning the actions taken, the Board of Trustees were irrevocably splintered, incapable of civility, and in dire need of supervision. Unfortunately, blocks of Trustees conspired to maintain control of the existing board and take action. Such a situation had been feared, forcing extraordinary actions on the part of the college community and the chiropractic profession.

In the initial salvo, the six Trustees who had been cited by the CCE were sent a petition signed by the student body requesting their resignations.[20] In the meantime, the administration, faculty and alumni continued working with attorneys to get the courts to intervene. In addition to the wheels of justice moving very slowly, it became apparent the courts did not wish to intervene in an educational matter, making the position of the college untenable. More radical action was needed.

On May 13, students walked out of school.

The administration, faculty, and alumni directly requested the State Department of Education and State Board of Regents intervene. Petitions signed by the members of the NYCC: administration, faculty and the alumni association, explaining the circumstances and requesting intervention had been submitted to the New York State Education Department.[21]

The following day, students rode to Albany on buses to meet with Donald Nolan, the deputy Director of the Department of Education, and explain their case. The officers of the Student Government met with the deputy commissioner and explained their frustration with how this conflict was adversely affecting their lives and future. Mr. Nolan recognized the gravity of the situation and agreed to address the Board of Trustees. On the basis of Mr. Nolan's willingness to address their issues, the students agreed to return to classes.[22]

On May 15, classes resumed and a degree or normalcy prevailed on campus.

At the next regularly scheduled faculty council meeting, May 17, the membership became aware of the agenda for the next Trustees meeting. Certain faculty members who were "friends" of board members had been given information on what was planned for the board meeting. These faculty members shared what they knew was about to happen at the board meeting, but they never anticipated the reaction of the faculty. There was no provision for the State Department of Education to be heard or conflict of interest issues to be addressed. On the agenda, the composition of the board and administration of the college was about to be altered. The outrage of the faculty, which had not been anticipated, occurred. The faculty voted to strike, immediately.

No classes were conducted the following day as students and faculty returned to Albany. The purpose of this trip was to meet with legislators, explain the circumstances they were looking to correct and request help. The efforts of the faculty and students were fruitful as many legislators wrote supportive letters on behalf of the college. Despite the letters sent to Chancellor Barrell of the Board of Regents, action by the Board of Regents was not forthcoming.[23]

The reconstituted trustees met on campus, on May 30. At lunch time the meeting was recessed and eight Trustees retired to Sage's restaurant in Mineola to have lunch. At this meeting, as anticipated, the Board of Trustees replaced Neil Stern as acting president with an individual by the name of Howard Genano, D.C. Frank Langilotti, in an apparent appointment to offset the academic inexperience of Dr. Genano, was named first Vice President of the college. Mr. Louis Wein replaced Mr. Vito Forte as Chairman of the Board, and Richard Carnival who had served on the board previously was re-appointed to the board.

It was apparent, with students boycotting classes, faculty striking, the college being in the news daily, and additional illegal action being taken by the board and reversed by the courts, the situation was spiraling out of control. On June 2, Judge Stuart Ain requested the State Board of Regents intervene in this deplorable situation.

The presidency of Howard Genano and Chairmanship of Louis Wein lasted one day as Justice Robert Roberto Jr. reversed the actions taken by the board and additionally enjoined the board from any further action. The same day, the State Board of Regents received petitions from Chairman Forte requesting their immediate intervention.

While Judge Ain requested intervention by the Board of Regents and Judge Roberto enjoined the Board of Trustees from future action, an additional audience became involved when the president of NYSCA and NYCC board member Robert Matrisciano, wrote a letter to the membership of the state trade association. In it he recounted the chronology of events that had transpired since the action taken by the CCE.[24]

On June 9, the Board of Regents agreed to conduct hearings on the Board of Trustees of the New York Chiropractic College. By the middle of June, after two months of campus unrest, the court-imposed stay remained in effect, the Board of Regents would be conducting hearings and classes had resumed.

While all this was transpiring, Rolla Pennell wrote a letter to the New York clients of Practice Masters wherein he listed seven points of contention which he "explained" to his clients.[25] Dr. Pennell's letter was cleverly constructed to describe the deceit that had been perpetrated on the students of the college, flavored by Dr. Pennell's perspective. The spin on his point of view was rebutted in a letter sent to Dr. Pennell by the administration, faculty, student body and alumni. In this rebuttal, each statement espoused by Dr. Pennell was offset by objective, factual information exposing his position as inaccurate.[26] The exchange of letters was an example of the futility of the situation. People, whether clients of Clinic Masters or members of the New York State Chiropractic Association were being informed of the unfortunate events occurring at the college and these people had no bearing on the final outcome of the case. On the one hand, Dr. Pennell was attempting damage control to maintain his stature with his clients by providing them with his side of the story. On the other hand, the response to Dr. Pennell's letter, which took hours to compose, was written and delivered, to potentially be entered into evidence, if additional court proceedings became necessary. After weeks of court room hearings and maneuvers, the Board of Regents had agreed to investigate the charges against and actions of the Board of Trustees of the New York Chiropractic College. The results of this investigation would prove who, in the eyes of the authorities, acted in the best interest of the college.

The Board of Regents Committee would render a decision after following a precise schedule to allow sufficient time to consider all the evidence. Hearings would be conducted. The testimony and exhibits of the court proceedings would be reviewed. Final written arguments submitted by the attorneys representing the Trustees were due July 31, and closing oral arguments were scheduled for August 15, 1986.

Despite the injunction of Judge Roberto prohibiting any action by the NYCC Board of Trustees, a meeting was scheduled for August 7 and 8, a week before closing oral arguments before the Regents' committee. The new officers of the NYCC Student Government had been approached by Louis Wein and Frank Langilotti in an attempt to foment unrest on campus. They wanted to get their "side" of the story to the student body. In what had been already discussed and planned, Dr. Langilotti was actively recruiting faculty to take teaching positions of faculty to be released after the meeting on August 7 and 8.[27] I was, most likely, on the list of individuals to be replaced. In addition to our longstanding personality conflict, Dr. Langilotti was also aware of a letter I had written to Dr. Stern when he had been criticized for the administration of the clinic exit examination.[28] This memo was composed and delivered approximately one month before Dr. Langilotti was appointed vice president by the Board of Trustees. In my letter to Dr. Stern, I recommended the repeal of the warm body and Billy Martin policies. The purpose of my letter was to illustrate Dr. langilotti had maintained his positions at the college based on these policies and not his ability. The insulting contents of the letter were also intended to incite Dr. Langilotti's temper. These same comments were a source of motivation for Dr. langilotti to succeed in his appointment as vice president. He could get even with me and impress his new benefactors on the Board of Trustees at the same time.

Trustees Forte, Matrisciano, Abruzzo and Bonetti were represented by the law firm of Liebowitz, Villanova & Royster.

Trustees Blake, Calton, Heuser, Pennell, Rousch and Zerdin were represented by Peter Costigan, Esquire.

Trustees Klein, Wein and Zoller were represented by Donald Shaw, Esquire.

The New York Chiropractic College paid the fees of all the attorneys representing the members of the board.

The Regents Committee investigating the NYCC Board of Trustees was chaired by Jorge Batista; and members included Shirley Brown and Laura Chodos. The final report numbered 30 pages and the findings of the committee were based upon 2,822 pages of testimony and nearly 200 exhibits. All the NYCC Trustees were questioned and cross-examined by the various attorneys involved.

The background of the controversy, as printed in the final Regents Committee report reads, "New York Chiropractic College is chartered by the Board of Regents and its educational program is registered with the New York State Education Department. That registration is the basis for the admission of graduates of the college to the practice of chiropractic in this state. The Council on Chiropractic Education is a national, private accrediting agency which evaluates and accredits the educational programs of colleges of chiropractic. Accreditation by the Council on Chiropractic Education is the basis for acceptance of educational programs for purposes of licensure in many other states. The program of the New York Chiropractic College is accredited by the Council on Chiropractic Education.

"The Council on Chiropractic Education has published formal educational standards for colleges of chiropractic which include standards for members of the Board of Trustees of such colleges. Those educational standards were formally adopted by the Board of Trustees of the New York Chiropractic College on December 4, 1977 and December 7, 1980."[29]

The report then went on to explain the confidential probation status that had been determined for NYCC as a result of the January 1986 meeting. The grounds stated for that resolution included a determination by the Commission "that several Trustees are in violation of the Standards Section III, subsection B. Organization, Item 1 Obligations, and Item 2. Responsibilities, specifically that Trustees receive no financial benefit from the operations of the college or from any other member or members of the board and administrative staff or from businesses or enterprises controlled or directed by them."[30]

Thee Regents Committee then reviewed the complicated maze of legal proceedings which had marred this situation from the beginning. The committee then stated, "The charges against the Trustees in this proceeding are based upon the provisions of Education Law, Section 226, subdivision 4, and the specifications of 'misconduct, incapacity, or neglect of duty' alleged in the petition, cross-petition and counter-petition.[31] We have based our recommendations on those charges and, in a few instances, on acts which were freely admitted by Trustees in their testimony, and which constitute misconduct." The report went on to say the committee did not consider additional acts or omissions even where, in the committees opinion, such acts or omissions could serves as the basis for additional charges.[32] The behavior of the Trustees under investigation was so outrageous and validated by evidence, no additional charges were warranted to substantiate the actions taken by the Board of Regents.

The cases of Gordon Heuser and Rolla Pennell were considered together. The report read, "Their business interests existed for many years and until on or about October 1, 1985, at which time Dr. Heuser transferred his interests to Dr. Pennell." The charges against the two included:

Misusing their positions as Trustees to lend credibility to products which were designed, manufactured or sold by their businesses;

Exercising undue influence over the conduct of research at the college in order to attempt to validate products which they sold, and to obtain approval by insurance companies of claims for the use of such equipment.

Misusing their positions as Trustees to obtain student lists and access to improper solicitation methods which were denied to their competitors.

Acting as Trustees to the detriment of the college and in favor of their business interests.

In all, there were seven separate charges considered by the committee which led to the recommendation,"Drs. Heuser and Pennell be removed from office as Trustees of the New York Chiropractic College."[33]

The committee recommended the charges against Dr. Mahlon Blake, Dr. William Rousch and Mr. Roger Calton be dismissed. In explaining the rationale behind their actions, the Regents Committee, in the matter of Mahlon Blake, refused to apply the strict interpretation of conflict of interest used by the Council on Chiropractic Education.[34] The Regents' Committee was not charged with interpreting and analyzing the CCE Standards, but New York State Education Law, Section 226, subsection 4. On that basis alone, the charges against Trustees Blake, Rousch and Calton were dismissed.[35]

Mr. Harold Zerdin used his position as a Trustee and his influence with the former president of the college to promote sales for businesses which he owned or with which he was associated, and that he intervened with the former president to prevent competition. All the charges made against Mr. Zerdin were sustained and it was recommended by the committee that he be removed from office as a Trustee of the New York Chiropractic College.[36]

The charges against Louis P. Wein were as follows:

Engaging in a commercial venture with Mr. Zoller in which they are listed on promotional material as trustees of the college;

Seeking to trade on his position as a Trustee for the benefit of the commercial venture;

Presenting the appearance of impropriety and of improper conduct in violation of Council on Chiropractic Education standards;

Acting in an irresponsible manner in the conduct of his office on and after March 1, 1986.[37]

The committee found that Mr. Louis Wein solicited funds from Trustees and from the acting president of the college for the organization of a commercial venture known as International Diagnostic Corporation (IDC). A prospective associate in that venture was Gerald Stephens, D.C., who had invested $50,000 and was named president of IDC. In testimony before the committee, Dr. Stephens testified that Mr. Wein had indicated if he and his associates lost control of the Board of Trustees at the college some of the Trustees would not invest in the company and IDC would not "get the diagnostic on board out of the school." Dr.

Stephens also shared the proposal, offered by Mr. Wein, to expand the size of the Board of Trustees by adding "safe votes."[38]

Evidence showed Mr. Wein also solicited investments from Trustees and college staff in another business in which he held stock, the Universal Satellite Corporation (USATCO).

In Mr. Wein's case, the bulk of testimony was offered by the president of IDC, Dr. Stephens. At the time of the Regent's Committee hearings Dr. Stephens was in private litigation against Mr. Wein.

The report read, "Mr. Wein was not one of the six Trustees found by the Council on Chiropractic Education to be in violation of its standards, and the evidence against him rests largely on the testimony of Dr. Gerald Stephens . We nonetheless conclude his testimony concerning Mr. Wein is credible and that the evidence establishes that Mr. Wein intended and attempted to use his influence as a Trustee to promote his personal business interests. The recommendation of the Regents Committee was Louis Wein be removed from office as a Trustee of the New York Chiropractic College."[39]

Louis Wein maintained an inflated opinion of his importance in this matter. He had developed a witness list of individuals to be examined during the hearings before Judge Suozzi. The schedule listed 37 individuals, including opposing attorneys, to be cross-examined over a period of three days. The names on the list were categorized as Trustees, NYCC Administration/Faculty, Students, and Others. Of interest on Mr. Wein's list were the names of Dr. Ed Epstein and Dr. Ken Padgett, neither of whom were directly associated with the college.[40] Because neither individual ever testified during the court proceedings, what information they could provide germane to the issues of conflict of interest was never uncovered. Several months later, both men were appointed to the Board of Trustees of the New York Chiropractic College.

The charges against Clifford Zoller, although substantiated in the evidence reviewed in the case of Mr. Wein, were dismissed.[41] The committee reported that Mr. Zoller's participation in the International Diagnostic Corporation was that of a passive investor. He did not use his position as a Trustee to actively promote the project.

A second Trustee who had not been identified by the Council on

Chiropractic Education as being in violation of their policy on conflict of interest, but cited in the committee reports, was Genevieve Klein. The charges against Mrs. Klein which were reviewed by the Regents Committee, were based upon her actions as a Trustee of the college and former member of the Board of Regents. It had been alleged Mrs. Klein attempted to intimidate the president of the NYCC student council by threatening licensure difficulties if he did not cease his activities with regard to the strife on campus. Furthermore, in extensive sworn testimony before Judge Suozzi, Mrs. Klein denied it was her voice on tape recordings of telephone calls to the president of the student council, but recanted that testimony at a later hearing.

The Regents Committee report characterized Mrs. Klein's testimony as, "at best, vague and evasive," and noted that during her testimony, Judge Suozzi cautioned her against committing perjury.[42]

The original charge against Mrs. Klein had been established but had been overshadowed by her effort to deny the phone conversation with the president of the student council. During this phone call, which was conducted under the guise of Mrs. Klein being the mother of a student, she attempted to dissuade the student council president from circulating a petition in opposition to the six trustees cited by the CCE. Her conduct on the phone, by refusing to give her name, and making guarded statements about licensure difficulties if he did not discontinue his activities were clearly improper conduct for a member of the Board of Trustees of the college. Her testimony before Judge Suozzi was characterized as even more serious.

By mailgram dated August 24, 1986, addressed to the Chancellor of the Board of Regents, Genevieve Klein resigned from the Board of Trustees of the New York Chiropractic College. As a result no further action was necessary by the Board of Regents.[42]

Counter-charges were made against Trustees Vito Forte, Salvatore Abruzzo, George Bonetti and Robert Matrisciano. These charges were focused on:

Trustees conspiring to and violating Education Law 226 (41) by illegally removing six members of the board from office:

    a.   By a vote of less than a majority of the full board'

b. Without a written complaint, due examination or proof of any misconduct, incapacity or neglect of duty,

c. Without notice of the proposed action;

Trustees having willfully and unlawfully deprived the six Trustees of their constitutional rights to a fair hearing and to due process of law;

Advising students, faculty and administrative staff to go on strike if the six Trustees did not resign;

Subjecting faculty, students and administrative staff to "pressures, threats of death, lies and other tactics to induce them to go out and stay out on strike."[43]

There is no reference in the Regents Committee report to the challenges faced by a minority segment of the board having to overcome a majority with potential ulterior, illegal motives. With so many votes aligned with Drs. Heuser and Pennell because of the similarity of interests between them and a majority of board members, the possibility of a fair, objective hearing, conducted by the full NYCC Board of Trustees was negligible. Unless some outrageous behavior occurred, such as boycotting classes, faculty strikes, and bus rides to Albany to get legislators involved, the outside intervention required to clean up the board would not have occurred. That was the rationale that motivated Trustees Forte, Bonetti, Abruzzo and Matrisciano.

Despite hearing testimony related to Mr. Wein wherein the expansion of the board with "safe votes" was a priority to maintain control of the board, the Regents Committee restricted their recommendations to the deviations of the four Trustees from the letter of the law. Even after Judge Ain re-constituted the board, which then named a new president and chairman—actions which were overturned by the court—the Regents Committee refused to comment on how their eventual involvement in the matter did not occur until after all the machinations caused by the "illegal" activities of the minority block of Trustees forced the situation.

The Regents Committee report read, "Prior to the March 1, 1986, board meeting, the college had a serious problem. After that meeting, it had a catastrophe."[44] With this statement the Regents Committee set the stage to remove Trustees Matrisciano, Bonetti, Abruzzo and Forte from office as Trustees of the New York Chiropractic College.[45]

The Regents Committee report concluded, "In the context of this situation at the college, we have concluded that the return of a sound educational environment and of a stable and effective leadership and management at the college can be accomplished only by the removal from office of nine of the Trustees, and the evidence and admissions justify their removal.

"We find that the actions of these Trustees constituted misconduct within the meaning of Education Law 226, subdivision 4, and that it is no longer in the educational interests of this college that they continue to serve as members of the Board of Trustees."[46]

Of the original group of Trustees identified by the Council on Chiropractic Education as having a conflict of interest which caused the New York Chiropractic College to be placed on confidential probation, the report of the Regent's Committee recommended the removal of three. The other six Trustees removed from office were found by the Regents Committee to have committed misconduct.

The Board of Regents replaced nine Trustees of the New York Chiropractic College with nine new Trustees, none of whom were chiropractors. The new Trustees were:

Benito Lopez, J.D.	Alceste T. Pappas, PhD
James J. Conte, PhD	Daniel Robinson, B.S.
Harry E. Ekblom, LL.B.	Stuart Steiner, J.D.
Allen T. Gittleson	Robert L. Werner, LL.D.
J. William Nystrom, PhD	

These individuals joined the other Trustees who had survived the intervention of the Board of Regents:

Mahlon Blake, D.C.	Roger W. Calton, J.D.
Nathan Novick, D.C.	William T. Rousch, D.C.
Winfield W. Salisbury, Sc.D.	Clifford Zoller

The Board of Trustees now consisted of 15 members, three of whom were chiropractors. The stage was set for the Board to influence the New York Chiropractic College and the profession of chiropractic moving into the future. [47]

In a letter to the Board of Trustees dated January 29, 1987, Acting President Stern reported "… by action of the Commission, the college has been *removed* from Confidential Probation and placed back in the normal cycle of accreditation."[48]

The conflict had finally been resolved.

Setting the Stage

The Board of Trustees' issues were corrected by the end of the summer. The next challenge for the newly constituted board was the selection of the new president. Unfortunately, the drama and chaos which had been evident throughout the resolution of the trustees' conflict[1] continued during the presidential search process.

Neil Stern, the acting president and a candidate for the presidency, was in the unenviable position of having been involved in the resolution of the trustees' issues. He also had the task of explaining chiropractic and college history to a board of trustees whose experience with chiropractic education was confined to the tumultuous cascade of events which lead to their appointment as trustees. Dr. Stern's involvement alienated him from at least four trustees who had been investigated by the Regents' Committee and allowed to retain their seats. His ascendency to the presidency would be a challenge. Not only were there at least four votes against him, he lost an additional four votes when trustees Abruzzo, Bonnetti, Forte, and Matrisciano were dismissed from office. During the court proceedings Bob Matrisciano, once believed to be the next president of the college, confided in me that he would support Neil Stern for the position. He felt his associates would also vote for Dr. Stern. The collateral damage of the Regents' Committee findings was the candidacy of Neil Stern.

Among other issues incumbent upon Dr. Stern was to explain the apparent lack of alumni support for the college. In a letter to trustee Lopez[2], Dr. Stern pointed out that when he graduated from the Columbia Institute of Chiropractic in 1968, he graduated with eight other students. (Dr. Stern would sometimes joke that he graduated in the top ten of his class). A review of the 1968 Columbian reveals 11 graduates and a student body which numbered less than 50 according to the pictorial information in the book.[3]

In his letter to trustee Lopez, Dr. Stern made several suggestions how to quell the fears and misapprehensions of college supporters about the new Board of Trusteees. Among the questions needed to be answered were: Who are these people?Where do they come from? What do they know about chiropractic? Why aren't there more chiropractors on the board? Will the next president be a D.C. or PhD? Will the next president understand chiropractic and the needs of the college? Will the next president be able to defend the principles of chiropractic against the incessant attacks of political medicine?

Throughout 1986 and 1987 Dr. Stern maintained a steady stream of correspondence with the members of the board. One of the first letters of correspondence between Dr. Stern and the then board chair, J. William Nystrom PhD, covered the NYIT – NYCC contract. In this same letter, Dr. Stern provided Chairman Nystrom with the terms of office of the trustees who had been retained after the actions taken by the Board of Regents. This information had been requested by the chairman.[4]

The issue of the New York Chiropractic College being a free-standing institution of higher and professional learning was a topic Dr. Stern pursued during his presidency and presidential candidacy. In a letter to Chairman Nystrom Dr. Stern referenced accreditation reports from the Council on Chiropractic Education and the Middle States Association which stated the need for the College to be free-standing.[5]

In a letter to the Board of Trustees, dated November 18, 1985 Dr. Stern started explaining how the budget process had been implemented at NYCC.[6] A year later, a follow-up report was submitted. By this time, expenditures and revenue were identified by line item. The rate of Bundy aid had risen to $4500. For each NYCC graduate receiving a degree. The anticipated revenue on this line item, in excess of $900,000, was based upon 222 students graduating.[7] Despite the distractions of the trustees' conflict, the administrative team overseeing the college, under the supervision and tuteledge of Neil Stern had been able to develop a more sophisticated budgetary process than the one submitted the previous year.

Chairman Nystrom resigned his office as a trustee and applied for the presidency. Dr. Nystrom's candidacy helped to motivate the development of a document titled, "The Case for Conflict of Interest."[8]

In this document, the actions taken by Dr. Nystrom were articulated for all the members of the Board of Trustees to consider.

An individual named Charles Nelson, a personal friend of Chairman Nystrom, was introduced to the Board of Trustees, then appointed, by the

Board, to head the search process for the new president. In this position, Mr. Nelson would screen applicants and advise the search committee which candidates were worthy of interviews.

Dr. Nystrom, as Chairman of the Board, appointed the chair and members of the search committee. One of the appointees was the president of the NYCC Faculty Council, Philip Striano, D.C., C.I.C.'67. The appointment of one vote to mollify the internal constituencies of the school would not change the ultimate decision made by the full committee.

Dr. Nystrom altered the College by-laws to allow original board members to continue in office for six months after their terms had expired. Whereas the Regents' Committee report had cost Neil Stern at least 8 votes, the system created by Chairman Nystrom ensured him a relatively easy path. Dr. Nystrom introduced his candidacy for president at the final meeting of the search committee.

Candidates for the presidency could have applied for the position on their own initiative or be nominated. The internal candidates interviewed by Mr. Nelson included Neil Stern, James McDonnell, Henry Shull, Louis Filardi and Frank Zolli. It is unclear how many external candidates were considered. By the time the process was nearing conclusion, the search committee had endorsed Jerome McAndrews D.C. for the position.

Dr. McAndrews was eminently qualified to be president having served as executive vice president of the International Chiropractors Association before becoming the president at Palmer College of Chiropractic (PCC). His presidency at Palmer lasted 8 years during which time he committed the institution to achieving regional accreditation. In addition, Dr. McAndrews initiated renovations to the college's physical plant to accommodate teaching the basic and clinical sciences. He also recruited a stable, full time faculty and initiated the first long – range planning process in the College's history. The McAndrews' administration at Palmer was committed to research and scholarly development. Jerome McAndrews had a proven record of academic achievement and integrity as a doctor of chiropractic and within chiropractic education.[9] He had demonstrated leadership and achievement in critical areas necessary for the development of the New York Chiropractic College.

The document sent to the Board of Trustees questioning the candidacy of Board Chair Nystrom, quoted, in part, the criteria listed in the advertisement for the presidency which had been printed in chiropractic and educational publications. Specifically quoted was he statement which read," The position requires an experienced person of unquestioned integrity, demonstrated educational leadership, strong management skills and a thorough knowledge of chiropractic, with the D.C. degree preferred." Jerome McAndrews fit the criteria listed perfectly.

The document concluded by asking the Board of Trustees two questions. Does J. William Nystrom possess these requirements? On what basis should he be the president of the New York Chiropractic College?[10]

Stuart Steiner, another Regents' appointee, succeeded Dr. Nystrom as chairman of the Board of Trustees. In a letter to his board colleagues he announced that Dr. Nystrom had acceded to the Board's request that he withdraw his resignation.Chairman Steiner continued,"However, because Dr. Nystrom has assumed significant new responsibilities in his position as vice president at Pace University he could not consider remaining as chair of the NYCC Board of Trustees.[11]

In February 1987 Benito Lopez was elected chairman of the Board of Trustees. Prior to Mr. Lopez being elected, Mr. Charles Nelson, the head of the presidential search process received a confidential letter from Jerome McAndrews withdrawing his candidacy for the presidency.[12]

In his letter, Dr. McAndrews he was concerned the immediate past chairman of the board had applied for the presidency. "There is a perception of ethical violations overshadowing the selection process." In addition to the past chairman's candidacy at the last minute, Dr. McAndrews indicated he had been advised he needed to talk to certain trustees to commit politically to certain sympathies or deny certain other affiliations if he hoped to "win" election to the presidency.

Finally he stated "appearances still exist that the Board of Regents' prior actions to clear the conflict of interest problem from the Board were incomplete or otherwise unsuccessful."[13]   Dr. McAndrews articulated what everyone on the NYCC campus and in the chiropractic profession was thinking, the NYCC Board of Trustees, whether assembled by Ernest G. Napolitano or by the Regents of the State of New York, could not seem to function in an ethical, professional manner.

The day after receiving Dr. McAndrews' letter, Mr. Nelson informed the Board of his decision.[14] As a result, the search was continued. The New York Chiropractic College and its various constituencies, which had been without a president since June of 1985, remained in limbo.

Four months later a press release was issued announcing the selection of Keith Asplin PhD as president of the New York Chiropractic College. In the same press release the election of 8 new members to the Board of Trustees was also announced. The press release followed the format that had been suggested by Dr. Stern in his letter to then board member Lopez.[15]

"In announcing these developments, Benito M. Lopez Jr., Chairman of the Board noted that the new president will assume his post in August 1987 and has long been involved in chiropractic education and is an experienced executive who will provide the leadership to make NYCC a major force in chiropractic education and research."[16]

Of the 8 new Board members, 5 were chiropractors. Edward A. Epstein, Chairman of the New York State Regents' Board for Chiropractic, Arnold Goldschmidt, President of the Federation of Chiropractic Licensing Boards, Martin Greenburg, former executive vice president of the New York Chiropractic College, Kenneth W. Padgett, member of the New York State Regents' Board of Chiropractic and Joanne Santiago, former president of the NYCC Alumni Association. According to the press release, 3 of the 5 new Board members were alumni of NYCC.[17] Both Dr. Epstein and Dr. Padgett had been listed as witnesses for Louis Wein during the trustees' debacle.[18] While their names on a witness list of a trustee who had been dismissed from office for misconduct do not indicate complicity on the part of either doctor in any type of unprofessional behavior, being elected to the Board at this time was questionable.

Upon the election of new trustees who were chiropractors, my position at the College was compromised. My association with Robert Matrisciano, a trustee who had been dismissed from office, was well known. We had spent hours together planning strategy with attorneys and in court waiting for legal proceedings to bear fruit. Dr. Matrisciano had won the presidency of the New York State Chiropractic Association (NYSCA) after a hard fought campaign against an upstate chiropractor and was seen by upstate chiropractors as a brash, arrogant Manhattan chiropractor. His management style was autocratic and similar to that of Ernest G. Napolitano. Despite his legislative victories which benefited chiropractors all over New York State, his upstate reputation was based upon fear. Dr. Matrisciano was feared and could no longer be touched. I was not and this was a chance to even the score and rid NYCC of any lingering connections to Ernest G. Napolitano.

The additional new Board members were J. Raymod Hinshaw, M.D. a member of the New York State Regents' Board for Medicine, Philip R. Johnston, former executive secretary of the New York State Regents' Board for Chiropractic and Helen Lowe, Vice President for Institutional Advancement at Marymount Manhattan College.

Gordon Heuser, D.C. was also elected to the Board, but declined the position.[19] Dr. Heuser was a former trustee who had been dismissed from office based upon the findings of the Regents' Committee. His re-election to the NYCC Board of Trustees, at this time, appeared questionable.

On the basis of these moves, the stage was set for the New York Chiropractic College to re-locate to upstate New York.

After being passed over for president, Neil Stern continued to work for the betterment of the college. He provided the Board of Trustees with proposed policies and procedures and became involved with short and long term planning.[20]

Citing conflict of interest based upon Dr. Raymond Hinshaw's political affiliations Dr. Stern objected to his election to the Board of Trustees. In his letter Dr. Stern reviewed the chronology of the Wilk Anti – Trust Case[21] and Dr. Hinshaw's involvement. He ended his letter by reminding Chairman Lopez that as a trustee and the head of the Board, he literally held, in trust, the fate of the college and, in part, the chiropractic profession.[22]

Throughout his term as interim president Neil Stern worked to improve the infrastructure at the New York Chiropractic College. Evidence of his commitment can be seen in a letter he wrote to the law firm of Sullivan and Cromwell in November 1986 wherein Dr. Stern requested a legal review a Conflict of Interest policy, a Trustee application, Proposed

By-Laws revisions, a Termination Policy, Contract proposals and Grievance Procedures. With the exception of revising the College By-Laws the
other policies and procedures had previously not existed at the college.[23]
On June 3, 1987 Dr. Stern wrote to trustee Nystrom requesting a review
by his subcommittee of an administrative grievance procedure and an
administrator's contract. Dr. Stern noted in this letter," members of the
administration have never had contracts."[24] Indirectly, Dr. Stern validated the futility of the threatened faculty strike in 1983. Dr. Napolitano
had read the commitment and the courage of the faculty accurately. He
reviewed the proposal which had been submitted, authorized a modest
increase in the pay scale, then let the balance of the proposal die, along
with the momentum and courage of the faculty. In the end he weathered
the storm of faculty discontent by making a token modification in the
pay scale and ignoring the other issues. His position as president and
power remained uncontested for the balance of his life.

Keith Asplin, PhD assumed office August 1, 1987. He had interacted
with Neil Stern previously when Neil had been the chairman of the
Commission on Accreditation and he represented Cleveland College of
Chiropractic – Los Angeles. Based upon these interactions there existed
an air of mutual animosity between the two. At the insistence of the
Board of Trustees, who recognized Dr. Stern's value to the institution,
Dr. Asplin made an unsuccessful effort at retaining Dr. Stern's services.[25]

By August when the Asplin administration began, Neil Stern had
accepted the position of Executive Vice President at Parker Chiropractic College (PCC). Parker had been granted recognized candidate for
accreditation status (RCA) by the Commission on Accreditation (COA)
of the Council on Chiropractic Education (CCE). The College was in the
process of securing accredited status. Who better than Neil Stern could
help Parker achieve accreditation? Dr. Stern had already sheparded the
New York Chiropractic College to accreditation with the CCE. He had
written the academic standards used by the Commission on Accreditation
in the evaluation process. He had been Chairman of the COA and was
well versed in the application and validation of the CCE accreditation
standards. He was also familiar with regional accreditation which would
be helpful when Parker sought accreditation from the Southern Associa-

tion of Colleges and Schools (SACS). Parker College of Chiropractic was CCE accredited in June 1988[26].

Based upon a review of records and correspondence from NYCC administrators, faculty, students and alumni, Dr. Asplin terminated the services of James McDonell, D.C. for "his negative personal influence and general incompetence."[27] Dr. McDonnell attempted to become involved in the North American College of Chiropractic initiative that was promoted sometime after he left NYCC.

To counter the anxiety created by these personnel changes, Henry Schull, D.C. was named head of academic affairs and Frank Zolli, D.C. assumed a similar position in student affairs.

Dr. Schull had been hired by acting president Stern in the spring of 1987. He had experience in curriculum development and brought a breadth of experience to NYCC that had previously not existed. Most importantly, he was an external hire. He was not an alumnus of the Columbia Institute of Chiropractic or NYCC. Dr. Schull was an alumnus of Palmer College of Chiropractic (PCC) and he had taught at both Palmer and Palmer –West chiropractic (PCCW) programs.

Additional appointments were made to the administration and for the first time regularly scheduled meetings were conducted between the administration and ad hoc committees of the Board of Trustees. These meetings should have been beneficial to both the College and the Board.

This first meeting was focused on long range planning. It was called to order by Chairman Lopez and attendees included trustees Ekblom, Novick, Robinson and Steiner, as well as President Asplin, Drs. Schull and Zolli and both a faculty and student observer.[28] President Asplin had met with Commission Chair Sullivan to discuss what was needed by NYCC to remain in compliance with CCE Standards. Dr. Sullivan indicated a functioning long range plan would be required by the January 1988 meeting. Dr. Sullivan also noted the history of non-compliance with CCE suggestions by the school could jeopardize the accreditation of the College.[29]

Board member Nathan Novick had been designated responsible for student affairs. An addendum to the minutes of the meeting indicated he had requested student comments be mailed directly to his home. Dr.

Novick was interested in student perceptions, positive or negative, of the administration, faculty, curriculum, facilities and student morale.[30]

At the next Board meeting, I was not informed of the student affairs committee meeting before the full Board meeting. An incomplete report was delivered to the full Board by Dr. Epstein, not Dr. Novick. The joint meetings to benefit the College were being used to undermine at least one member of the administration.

Dr. Asplin was in a position where he needed to provide leadership to the College while simultaneously demonstrating the character and decision making skills that would assure the Board they had made the right decision selecting him as president. After severing ties with Drs. Stern and McDonnell, and appointing Drs. Schull and Zolli, he made additional appointments. His plan was to monitor the progress made by his administrative team as it addressed the needs of the College. Unfortunately, he did not realize he had inherited a staff and infrastructure that was just starting to mature. It soon became apparent the growing pains required during the maturation process would undermine his plan.

The research efforts of the College were headed by Gerald Leisman, PhD, who was described by Dr. Asplin as an effective program administrator. What Dr. Asplin failed to realize was there was no infrastructure in place to support Dr. Leisman's initiatives. The faculty were not trained in research methodology. They did not understand the scientific method. They did not appreciate the need for research. In fact, the faculty resented research being performed on chiropractic. In their minds, chiropractic worked, why does it have to be proven? While Dr. Leisman was interested in performing research and securing grant money to support his initiatives, the culture of the faculty needed to be radically changed. This was a time consuming process that would require years to accomplish.

Paul Cadolino, D.C. was charged with supervising the Division of External Affairs. His primary responsibility was developing postgraduate and continuing education programs to compliment the undergraduate professional program. In an effort to support continuing education, his added responsibilities included alumni affairs, public relations and development. Each of these offices required an experienced professional to develop and maintain. Dr. Cadalino's qualifications were that he was an

NYCC graduate and he wanted to work in chiropractic education. The development of the Division of External Affairs was a failure. As a result the offices of alumni affairs, public relations and development were transferred to the Division of Student Affairs. The office of postgraduate and continuing education was transferred to the Division of Academic Affairs.

In the spring of 1988 the oversight of the registrar's office was transferred to the Division of Student Affairs. The shuffling of responsibilities was a time honored tradition at NYCC. Instead of recognizing a problem and employing a trained, experienced professional to correct the deficiency, the responsibilities were transferred to another administrator. When chiropractic was isolated from the general academic community this tactic may have been necessary, but now that progress had been made in achieving accreditation and correcting some of the misperceptions about chiropractic education, there was no reason for it to continue.

In the summer of that year the Board of Trustees had arranged for Dr. Asplin to attend an executive training course at Harvard University. He was absent from campus for six weeks. During that time the daily administration of the College was the responsibility of Dr. Schull. After this assignment ended, relations between personnel in the Divisions within the College and the president's office began to deteriorate.

Every day Dr. Asplin was at Harvard, Dr. Schull sat in the president's chair and answered the mail. Some external pieces of mail were deferred to Dr. Asplin, while internal correspondence was answered by Dr. Schull whose communication skills, if and when used, were abrasive.

In spring of 1989, I was a member of a CCE site team visiting Palmer College of Chiropractic. Prior to my leaving campus Dr. Asplin indicated he would need my phone number to ensure he would be able to contact me while I was away. I thought this was an odd request because on other occasions when I was away on site team visits a similar request had never been made. When I inquired why, Dr. Asplin assured me it was "just in case" he needed to talk to me.

On the first day of the Palmer site team visit, I called my office at NYCC to check on campus events. My secretary answered the phone. She was crying. When I asked her what was wrong, she advised me Dr. Asplin had just addressed an assembly of students, faculty and staff and announced NYCC was moving to a campus in upstate New York.

Élaine, you just don't move a college lock, stock and barrel."

That's what he said."

"Are there any other good rumors?," I inquired.

My secretary again started to cry, "You were fired."

"That might be true," I responded, "put me through to the president's office."

The phone was picked up immediately. "Good" morning I attempted to say when I was interrupted, "He wants to talk to you." I waited for a second on the phone untill heard a familiar voice say, "We're moving!" I didn't respond. "What do you think?" "I think we need to talk," was my response. The balance of the conversation was brief and addressed issues of no real importance. Between my shock and anger I wasn't interested in anything I was hearing. By the time the call had ended, we had agreed to meet when I returned to campus.

On July 1 of the previous year I had signed a three year contract with the College. Dr. Asplin had spoken with me and indicated my services to the college were valuable. He indicated the Board of Trustees wanted me to come on staff-full time. I had always maintained a private practice, Tuesday and Thursday afternoon and Saturday. Now I would be totally dependent on the College as the source of my income. After considering all of the ramifications of the offer and discussing the matter with my wife, I agreed. My decision was based, in part, by the College residing in Long Island. I lived a scant six miles from campus and family resided all over Nassau County. This proposed move was never part of the equation.

When I walked into the meeting with Dr. Asplin, the dialogue was direct and professional. "Keith, this didn't just happen. This move was being negotiated when you and were talking about my coming on full time here." He didn't dispute what I said. "We can do this nice or nasty, it makes no difference to me," I said, "but if we cannot agree on a severance package, I will sue the College." In May 1989 I submitted my letter of resignation to Dr. Asplin after working out a severance package I thought was fair. I left NYCC on June 30, one day shy of my one year anniversary of being a full – time employee.

Dr. Asplin wrote a letter to the Board of Trustees titled, "History of Staff Decisions at NYCC."[31] In it he attempted to explain how the Asplin administration had imploded. By the time this letter had been written my resignation had been accepted and was common knowledge on campus. It was also common knowledge Henry Schull would be leaving. The letter simply stated each of us would be replaced.[32] Dr. Asplin did note the need for experienced individuals to assume the administrative responsibilities of maintaining the campus to which NYCC would be re –locating.

On my last day on campus, I noticed an oil painted portrait of Ernest G. Napolitano in the garbage. I retrieved it along with a significant amount of chiropractic memorabilia. I donated some of the memorabilia to Cleveland College of Chiropractic, which houses a treasure of chiropractic history. After Frank Nicchi D.C. assumed the presidency of NYCC, I donated some artifacts to NYCC.I was confident Dr. Nicchi would respect the heritage of the College. Today this oil painting of Nappy hangs in the dean's conference room at the University of Bridgeport – College of Chiropractic.

Traditional chiropractic thought prevails that the head of a chiropractic program should be a chiropractor. Despite working in chiropractic education for years, the initials after Keith Asplin's name are PhD. As a result he became expendable as president as soon as a viable D.C. became available. That individual was reported in the same press release that announced Dr. Asplin's selection as president[33]. Board member Kenneth W. Padgett, D.C., a former president of the American Chiropractic Association (ACA) and member of the New York State Regents' Board for Chiropractic was waiting in the wings.

Opportunity

My career as an academician was over. The first day of retirement was a day of golf and contemplation. I enjoyed treating and helping patients, therefore my career choices were limited to the practice of chiropractic. My options for where to practice were wide open. I had secured licenses to practice in New Jersey and New York and had practiced in both locales. I had opened my practice in Jersey City, New Jersey, and actively treated patients, from February 1980 through June 1988. I had also practiced in Oceanside, Long Island, with two partners between 1982 and 1985. I liked practicing in Jersey, but the commute could be a hassle. I didn't like practicing in New York for a variety of reasons, some professional and some personal. Another option would be to bide my time, and possibly associate in an established practice.

The first order of business was to work on my golf game. I went to the Oyster Bay golf course and played 18 holes in the morning, then returned home. I wasn't in the house 30 minutes when the phone rang.

"Hello."

"How would you like to start a new chiropractic school?"

"Well, I have plenty of time on my hands right now."

"With your experience, this school could be great! Plus, this school will be part of a university."

"Wait a minute, what university would be willing to start a chiropractic school?"

"The University of Bridgeport."

My interest piqued, I then asked, "Are you serious?"

"Yes. They want to start a chiropractic program and they don't have anyone who knows anything about chiropractic to do it."

"Let me think about it and I'll get back to you. When do you need to know?"

"Well, there are a couple of other people I could call."

"My question was, when do you need to know my answer? Now, my next question is, are these other people you might be calling as good as me?"

"Not really."

"Good, then wait until you hear from me before you call them."

I hung up the phone. My mind was racing. Dropped in my lap is was the chance to start a chiropractic school. A school which will be part of an established university—a first for the chiropractic profession!

As a member of the administration of the New York Chiropractic College, I was aware of the pro-chiropractic history of the University of Bridgeport. One of the first undergraduate pre-chiropractic programs was initiated at UB. Dr. Napolitano had reached an agreement with UB to start a human nutrition program to provide chiropractors with training and an academic credential in nutrition. The University of Bridgeport had a proven record of cooperating with the chiropractic profession on academic issues. On the basis of the information I had, this opportunity appeared to be something worth pursuing.

I did not consider my lack of experience within a university could be problematic in carrying out my responsibilities. As a student I attended St. Peter's College in Jersey City. My professional education started at the Columbia Institute of Chiropractic and was completed at the New York Chiropractic College. I was aware that multiple academic programs made my undergraduate training complex. On a professional level, every aspect of training was focused on chiropractic. As a result, functioning in a university environment could be a culture shock. I would now have to share facilities and support services with other schools and colleges. I would now have to fight for funding during the annual budget process. At NYCC as a student, faculty member or administrator, if I needed to meet with anyone (except Dr. Napolitano), the meeting was scheduled and occurred quickly. I expected a similar set-up at UB. I was wrong.

Prior to starting work at the University of Bridgeport I had several meetings with the College of Chiropractic Committee members. It was explained to me that the University could not financially support the program.All funds were to be raised by the Committee.The plan was to solicit funds from the chiropractic profession. My job was to do everything else.

A press release issued by the University dated October 20, 1989, announced the Board of Trustees had approved proceeding with a planning process to establish a College of Chiropractic. In the press release several members of the UB administration and faculty were quoted, all of whom expressed positive sentiments about the venture.[1] Despite the positive comments expressed, I soon found out reality on campus was quite another thing.

(The following are excerpts from my diary. For information in my diary requiring further explanation, the italicized wording within the parenthesis after the diary entry will provide the reader with additional information.)

10/25/89–The first day. I awoke early, kissed my wife Happy Birthday and left for the university. I stopped at Bud Passero's to pick up a copy of the floor plan of the nursing building. This was the facility which had been vacated by the nursing program and designated to house the College of Chiropractic. I also received a copy of documents which had been presented to the Board of Trustees. On top of the regulations for licensure and accreditation was a memo from Dr. Eigel to Dr. Passero which read in part, "I will be in touch with you by phone to set up a meeting with whomever you suggest after you have had a chance to review this material."[2] I realized after receiving this information that I was the "whomever you suggest," referred to in the memo.

(Marino "Bud" Passero is a Connecticut chiropractor. He is also a chiropractic activist, serving the profession in numerous roles during his career. He has been involved in politics, education and professional relations, assuming highly influential roles in every area of his involvement on state, national, and international levels. He is the cousin of Carmen Tortora, a trustee at the University of Bridgeport. In the press release of October 20, Dr. Passero, a UB alumnus was identified as initiating discussions on the project with President Greenwood approximately six months prior to the announcement. Approximately six months would place the start of negotiations with the university in March. If negotiations with the university began in March, discussions on the project and planning for fundraising had to begin at the same time. With the project starting today, money to support the program should have been available.)

Went to the office I had been assigned, room 21 at Halsey Hall, 491 University Avenue, Bridgeport, Ct. Settled in, unpacked my belongings, reviewed some university material and the documents I had received from Bud. I then went to the bookstore.

When I returned to the office I received a call from a prospective student inquiring about admission to the new program.

(*At this time there was no chiropractic program, only a Chiropractic College Committee to aid in planning and development. The University could not advertise the program because it was not yet licensed by the state. As a result, the university or its representatives could not initiate contact with individuals to discuss the program. Representatives of the university could answer questions about the program, only after contact was initiated with us.*)

I plan on meeting with Ed Eigel today to discuss the steps necessary for licensure, CCE accreditation and regional accreditation. (*Dr. Edwin Eigel was the Provost of UB. He had sought the Presidency of the University when Janet Greenwood was selected as president. He was a mathematics professor who eventually succeeded Janet Greenwood as president, after she left the university*). The balance of the day was spent on writing the purposes and objectives of UBCC. I received keys for the front door and office.

10/30–I spent the morning working on information for the licensure proposal. There isn't a lot of activity on the UB campus on Mondays. I spoke with Ed Eigel and made an appointment for next Monday. He wants to review information with me that he received in Hartford. Called Mike Bisciglia (*Vice President of University Relations*) who was at a meeting and would not be getting back to me today. Called Bud Passero who advised me that as of today, one check, his, had been received. It had been explained to me prior to accepting this position that the University of Bridgeport could spend no money on this venture. All money that would fund this program would be raised by the Chiropractic College Committee. My acceptance of this position was based on an understanding I had with the committee members. I would do the planning, the writing of the reports, and providing all the work required to get the program licensed and accredited. They would raise the funds. At the appropriate time, a highly visible individual within the profession would assume the position of dean of the college. That person was never identified by any of the committee members, but it was clear, the person would not be me. I would remain a member of the administration of the program, just not the dean. I see my participation in this undertaking as a learning experience which will pay dividends in the future.

My experience up to this point in time has been restricted to nine years of administrative work at the New York Chiropractic College. This is a chance to learn how a university functions. Little did I realize my exposure to higher education had little to do with education. It would nonetheless be an education – in life.

(*The Chiropractic College Committee consisted of Arnold Cianciulli, D.C., (New Jersey) Robert Matrisciano, D.C., (New York), Marc Peyser, D.C. (Connecticut) and myself. Drs. Cianciulli, Matrisciano and Peyser had the responsibility of raising the funds to support the college.*

Arnold Cianciulli was a New Jersey chiropractor who was politically active. He was the driving force responsible for having progressive pro-chiropractic legislation passed in the New Jersey legislature. He was an appointee to the New Jersey Board of Medical Examiners He was also nationally involved in chiropractic politics as a member of the Board of Governors of the American Chiropractic Association. He had also served as an adjunct faculty member at NYCC, being a signer of the petition which had been submitted to the New York State Education Department at the start of the Trustees' crisis.

Robert Matrisciano was a New York chiropractor, who, as president of the New York State Chiropractic Association, was instrumental in having pro-chiropractic legislation passed in New York. He was responsible for having legislation passed allowing students at the New York Chiropractic College to use human cadavers for the study of anatomy. As a result of this legislation, the New York Chiropractic College, of which he was a Trustee, was able to complete plans and construct a state of the art anatomy facility to compliment the construction of its academic center. When I was a student at the Columbia Institute of Chiropractic, my anatomy training was conducted on rhesus monkeys. My girlfriend at the time, an art student at Pratt Institute, every Saturday morning would travel to the human anatomy laboratory at Columbia University to sketch human cadavers. It was illegal for me, a student of chiropractic to study from human cadavers, but it was legal for artists to study using cadavers.

Marc Peyser was an up-and-coming chiropractic activist in the state of Connecticut. As a student at the Columbia Institute of Chiropractic he had been used as a model in Frank DeGiacomo's book on palpation. These three individuals had the visibility, pedigree and connections to reach out and raise money. Each of them were directly connected with the New York Chiropractic College, which had moved away.

After six months of planning, one check had been received! Obviously the committee members were not promoting the project nor soliciting funds.)

I had a meeting with Jackie Benamati *(UB Director of Admissions)* to discuss admission criteria and campus housing. Upon my return to the office I received a call from Bud Passero who outlined a plan for fundraising to start immediately. A second phase would begin in January.

(Fundraising was to begin immediately, after six months of "negotiating." It was my belief the fundraising plan had been well thought out. It should have been started by the time I started work on the project. The members of the committee all had experience in politics. They all had experience in funding projects that required support throughout the duration of the initiative. Although I had not worked closely with everyone on the committee, I knew each of them by reputation. Each member of the committee had produced successful results throughout their careers. Although I was disappointed to find out that fundraising was just beginning, I was comforted in knowing a second phase had already been determined.)

11/6–Spent the day working on licensure application. I spoke with a chiropractor from Connecticut, who had called regarding a faculty position. I also spoke with a prospective student. I put in a call to Mike Bisciglia who is on vacation until 11/20/89. I received a résumé from another Connecticut D.C. who wants to be part of the new program. I spoke with a NY chiropractor who was a former student of mine. He indicated he would contribute a couple of thousand dollars to the project. I spoke with Bob Matrisciano who indicated he was holding a couple of checks. He also indicated he did not know what was going on with Bud or Arnold in terms of fundraising. The creation of the College of Chiropractic is not a new initiative, yet financial planning is way behind schedule. I believe the intentions of the Chiropractic College Committee are good, but I do not understand their reluctance to financially support this project. In addition to the external challenges of raising money, we are not used to the bureaucracy that is the university. If the committee wanted to sponsor a fund raising event it needs to be co-ordinated through special events. We are no longer at NYCC, a small school where things can get done at the last minute. Here, in this environment, everything requires planning- and time.

(I recognized the University of Bridgeport could not fund the chiropractic program at all. Funding would come exclusively from money raised by the Chiropractic College Committee. What surprised me was the lack of coordination between the Committee and the Development Office of the University. It seemed to me an office which raises money on a regular basis would be helpful in aiding a committee of professionals with no fundraising experience. I was more troubled by the apparent lack of communication by committee members with Bob Matrisciano. Dr. Matrisciano had access to the state with the largest number of chiropractors in the northeast. It didn't make sense to me that he would not be part of the planning process. He should be aware of the current plan and the next phase to start in January, yet he knew about neither.)

11/8–Work on the licensure project continues. I am hoping to submit the final copy to the provost tomorrow. I have yet to hear from Dr. Eigel this week, although his secretary keeps telling me he wants to talk to me. So far we have yet to connect. I have not heard from any members of the Chiropractic College Committee. I received another call from a Connecticut D.C., who wants to be involved in the project. I had received his résumé previously and outlined the process we would be following. I also received an inquiry from a faculty member, an associate professor of clinical sciences at Parker College. I wonder if Neil Stern *(VP at Parker College of Chiropractic)* knows this guy is looking to leave Parker; I wonder if he is any good?

I received a blind carbon copy of a letter Jackie Benamati sent to a variety of university personnel regarding the inquiry cards that will be used to track calls requesting information about the chiropractic program. This is the first time I have seen any kind of work turned around in a week's time. Hopefully this will start to generate some outside enthusiasm for the project. A small article appeared on the front page of *Dynamic Chiropractic* newspaper today, announcing the intentions of the university to move ahead with a chiropractic college. Again, I hope it is a source of positive enthusiasm for the project. It is now 5:30 PM and my typewriter has run out of ribbon, so I will close up shop for the day and work at home.

11/9–Made copies of all the information I have accumulated. I will give this information to the Chiropractic College Committee on Tuesday evening. I also submitted a copy to Ed Eigel for his review. I stopped at public relations to pick up a copy of the consultant's report I gave them a month ago. I asked Catherine Yang *(comptroller/associate vice president of finance)* for a copy of the floor plans for the nursing building, Dana Hall, and the library. With this information, the licensure application should be completed by Monday. The next step will be to contact the Council on Chiropractic Education (CCE) to start that ball rolling.

11/13–Got to the office to find that the information to answer the last question on the licensure application remains home. I busied myself accumulating the background information for exhibits which will need to be submitted along with the narrative. Catherine Yang gave me the information I requested last week, but indicated Dean Blackshaw was upset I had requested it. *(G. Lansing Blackshaw, was Dean of the College of Engineering at that time. He would later become the provost at UB before moving to the same position at the New York Chiropractic College).* She asked if I would meet with him and discuss my intentions with the floor plans. Dean Blackshaw and I met and discussed the program for about half an hour. His main concern was that Dana Hall was being renovated and if there were special needs the College of Chiropractic required, those revisions should be made now to the floor plans. The federal government had given the university a grant of $4 million for the renovation of this building. In typical university inefficiency, the money was used before the entire building had been renovated, which benefited the chiropractic program. When the time came for the College of Chiropractic to expand, the space available in Dana Hall accommodated the needs of the college.

(One thing I learned working within the university, everyone needs all of the space allocated to their program. If space becomes available adjacent to space used by their program, they need the available space. Space is a commodity in higher education that is maintained more dearly than life, and it is never given away.)

I finally had a chance to speak with Ed Eigel who indicated we would need to talk about the information I had submitted to him. He also asked if I had had stationery made. I indicated I had not and needed to speak with Mike Bisciglia regarding how to requisition stationery and equipment. I also stated that there must be forms I need to fill regarding payroll. He told me to meet with Mike and get back to him if there were any problems. I called Mike Bisciglia's office and made an appointment with him for Monday 11/20/89 at noon. The meeting is tentative. On Thursday I need to submit a copy of the curriculum to Dean Blackshaw and the last question for licensure to Ed Eigel. The balance of the day will be spent finishing the application to have ready for tomorrow night's meeting.

(*On November 15, 1989, a front page article in Dynamic Chiropractic announced the start of the process to establish a college of chiropractic at the University of Bridgeport. Unfortunately there was no coordination of this newspaper article with the fundraising campaign that was supposed to have started.*)

11/20–Completed licensure application. I will submit it to Ed Eigel on Wednesday.

11/22–To date only a couple of checks have been received, plus I have one. I can only hope more are received soon. I spoke with several more prospective students today, as well as a prospective faculty member. It seems funny, there is more interest being generated by prospective students than by the chiropractic profession.

11/23–Meeting with Mike Bisciglia at 10:30. I gave him $7500 in checks, as well as Bob Matrisciano's résumé. He is to be placed on the Board of Trustees. The licensure application was delivered to Ed Eigel. A lot of calls to make, including one to the NYCC student newspaper.

(*Meetings at the University are difficult to schedule. My original call to schedule a meeting with Vice President Bisciglia was October 30, 1989. It required almost a month to sit down and meet with him. It is more difficult to schedule a meeting with a member of the UB administration than it was to meet with Dr. Napolitano. While I understood the machinations of Nappy's scheduling process I think academic administrators at UB cannot be distracted by too many issues simultaneously.*)

The meeting with Mike Bisciglia went well. We spoke, then I ordered business cards, stationery and requisitioned a check for myself, finally. Hopefully, I will be paid next week.

11/29–No heat in building today.

12/4–Still no heat. Made an appointment with Eigel for 12/6 regarding licensure application. Submitted another check to Mike Bisciglia who informed me I will be getting a check on Wednesday. Spoke with Bud/Arnold; spoke with Bob (Matrisciano) on Friday. He is the only committee member soliciting funds for the program. Bud and Arnold are waiting for the brochure to be published, which I believe is a mistake. However it is difficult to tell these guys where their thinking may be deficient. Hopefully, in short order we should have $20,000 raised by Bob, which should keep the wolves from the door.

(At this point in time, I had raised more money ($2500) for the project than most of the members of the Chiropractic College Committee. The idea for a fundraising brochure was decided upon one evening at dinner at Il Bochetto, a restaurant located in the Bronx. The location of the restaurant was convenient to Manhattan, New Jersey, Connecticut and Long Island and we met there often. The idea for a brochure sounded good and raised the enthusiasm of the committee members, but in terms of its desired results, was a dismal failure.)

12/6–Got in the office to find the heat had just been turned on. Calls/interest generated from five more prospective students, bringing the total to date to 26.

While driving to school I was considering information I had received regarding an established school (National/New York) approaching the university about taking over its fledgling chiropractic program. This would give either school an edge in the east and solve NYCC's dilemma about moving to Seneca Falls. NYCC could move as far north as Bridgeport and inhabit dorms already in existence and ready for occupants. This could increase NYCC's northeast presence and allow them to attract students from across the country. The possibility is both intriguing and scary. The meeting with Eigel went well. There are a minimal number of revisions needed prior to submission which is scheduled for early January. I need to meet with the head of graduate admissions and the registrar's office to update information in the licensure application. Got a call from Mike Bisciglia's office. I am supposed to be paid on Friday.

12/8–Red letter day at UB–received half the money I was supposed to receive and was told by Mike Bisciglia that Bud (Passero) would have to tell him when to release the balance of the money. I called Bud and asked him to release the money this week and he informed me that Arnold had told him it was okay to release half the money owed to me this month and half next month. Furthermore, I would be taking less money because I would be working on the project only one day per week. I told him I had never agreed to that. He told me he would have to get back to me.

(*This was the first time I became aware that the university was not in charge of the chiropractic program, it was under the control of Dr. Passero, who was being advised by Dr. Cianciulli. I had been living on the severance payment I had received when I left NYCC. Monthly payments and normal expenses were being addressed, but I needed to offset these payments with a regular stream of revenue. Communication between myself and the members of the committee was by no means regular and I resented these men making decisions for the program and myself and my family without so much as a courtesy call for my input. This situation confirmed what I had suspected about the Chiropractic College Committee and why communication with Bob Matrisciano was lacking.*)

12/11–Met with Barbara Gabianelli, the university registrar regarding what needs to be done with the school. I also met with Lucy Marini regarding graduate admissions to get that process on track. I spoke with Bob, Arnold and Bud regarding our meeting tomorrow night. Bud admitted it was a matter of money holding things up. I told Bob we need to take the bull by the horns and get the thing moving.

(*The first phase of fundraising which was to start "immediately" in October had not yet started*).

12/15–Spent the morning talking with prospective students and writing press releases. I will not be getting paid today–what a surprise. I am supposed to be paid on Monday. It is also the day I will be submitting my next pay voucher.

I spoke with Arnold this morning. He loved the press releases, but when I asked him about the timetable for the program starting, he got defensive.

(*Since the first phase of fundraising was to start in October and was two months late, and the second phase had not even been discussed, the fundraising campaign to support this initiative was looking worse than I could have imagined. By now I would have been practicing laying a foundation for my future instead of anguishing about issues which were supposed to have been addressed.)*

1/8/90–It has been some time since my last entry. Things have been very slow. The university is closed for another week. The number of calls coming in have been minimal. However, at this time, we have inquiries from 40 students and 18 faculty.

Our first press release appeared in the *ACA Journal*. Arnold indicated the articles I submitted to Don Peterson Jr. will be getting printed. Bob Matrisciano wants me to check out holding a continuing education seminar at the university. I have to contact the State of Florida and see what arrangements have to be made at the university. Spoke briefly with Ralph Miller (*Executive Director of the CCE*) about starting the process for professional accreditation.

1/10–Got in the office today to find a front page article about UB in the *Chiropractic Journal*. It was a verbatim copy of the press release distributed by the university. I also received two more faculty inquiries, one from an individual I have spoken to several times and the other from a D.C. in Florida. The Florida D.C. kept referring to the program as chiropractic medicine.

There has been little or no fundraising activity in a long time. I hope it starts soon.

I spoke with Ralph Miller again about the CCE accreditation process. Ralph suggested we hold off for a couple of weeks until after the January meeting of the CCE so that the new standards would be in force and clarified.

I ordered covers for the licensure application from Mike Bisciglia's office.

1/12–Minor disappointment today. Lillian Nash who was good enough to agree to type the licensure report has been unable to complete the assignment. I'm hoping to get it completed by Monday. *(Lillian Nash was the secretary in the office the Vice President of Finance. She is a longtime employee of the University of Bridgeport who eventually became the Administrative Assistant to the Provost).*

I called Jean Southard about my check and she indicated it will be ready sometime today. Just my luck, I will be leaving early today, so I'll have to pick it up on Monday. (*Jean Southard was the Director of Accounts Payable for the University*). *She functioned in a highly stressful position, talking daily with vendors owed money by the university. As the financial condition of the University deteriorated, her job became progressively more difficult.*)

Hopefully the wording of the bylaws Arnold has produced with Ed Harkin (*Arnold's friend and attorney*) will be acceptable to the Board of Trustees so that some effective fundraising can get going.

(*Dr. Cianciulli had indicated his reluctance to raise funds for the project was the lack of a written agreement between the university and the Chiropractic College Committee regarding the proposed program. Obviously this reluctance was shared by Dr. Passero, but never discussed with Dr. Matrisciano. It was also never discussed with me. In all of my meetings with the members of the Chiropractic College Committee the lack of a written agreement between the committee and the University was never cited as an issue impeding the fund raising process.*)

1/15–Licensure application completed, only requires review/ grammatical edits. Met with Ray Wiegans D.C. to discuss putting computer program into our curriculum. This may be good opportunity to put UBCC on the cutting edge of chiropractic research/information technology.

I hope to have the completed licensure application to Ed Eigel by 1/17/90, after which we can attack the balance of the program.

The completed licensure application was hand delivered to the provost's office at 4:00 PM on 1/15/90. Now we wait and see.

A second newspaper article announcing the start of the process of establishing a chiropractic program at the University of Bridgeport appears in the Chiropractic Journal. Without coordination to a fundraising campaign the results were predictably negligible.)

1/17–Mail this morning from Bob Matrisciano, a student inquiry and several faculty résumés. At present we have 57 student inquiries. I hope the fundraising brochure goes out soon. We need to pursue the interest generated in the program so far with credible evidence that this project is alive.

I received information today from Iso Technologies about a back testing machine. I replied asking for more information. I hope to incorporate this unit (as a donation) into some solid research in the cost effectiveness of chiropractic care.

1/19–We have now exceeded 60 student inquiries. More faculty inquiries are also being generated. Still waiting to hear from Eigel.

Spoke with Marc Peyser today about the program. He is looking for the establishment of this school to help the political efforts of the Connecticut Chiropractic Association.

(Marc Peyser, at this point in time, assumed a more active role on the Chiropractic College Committee. Dr. Passero would be assuming a seat on the Council on Chiropractic Education. As a result, his involvement with a particular chiropractic program would not be prudent.)

Things are happening in New York. In addition to the New York State Chiropractic Association and the Empire State Chiropractic Association, two new organizations have emerged. The newest groups are the Federated County Societies of New York and the New York Chiropractic Council.

(The New York State Chiropractic Association, had prospered under the leadership of Bob Matrisciano. Dr. Matrisciano was not afraid to initiate lawsuits or fight against any agency posing a threat to the chiropractic profession. His attitude and actions were a source of discomfort to some members of the profession, but everyone in the profession in New York enjoyed the benefits of his legislative accomplishments. He had hosted a fundraiser for Governor Mario Cuomo, which the governor attended, and raised an impressive amount of money to aid in chiropractic lobbying efforts. The political prominence of the chiropractic profession under Dr. Matrisciano was poised to continue and grow, but after serving two terms as president, he retired from office. The organization after his retirement was unable to maintain the momentum of positive achievement and the aggressive attitude which was required to make progress. The inability of NYSCA to provide leadership and results for chiropractors in New York in subsequent administrations opened the door for other state trade associations, and further depleted the limited resources and morale of chiropractors in the state.)

1/22–Interviewed for channel 12 cable television network (Norwalk). The program is supposed to be on this evening.

Still waiting to hear from Eigel.

1/24–Walked in this morning to rave reviews. Lillian Nash indicated the news network did about a three minute piece on the university. I received a call from a D.C., M.D. who wants to teach in the program in addition to several résumés of UB faculty who want to be affiliated with the chiropractic program.

I turned over a check to the university. The Executive Committee of the Board of Trustees is scheduled to meet, I figured it would be good for the board to see money being generated by the program.

1/26–The weather for the past 48 hours has been dreadful, rain drizzle, rain miserable. I hope things get better.

The *NEWSLETTER*, the AAUP communication device came out today with an article entitled, "Six Reasons Why UB Should Not Start a Chiropractic Program."

The article was written by a faculty member of the law school. I called Sheila Burke and asked her about the publication. She indicated it was standard fare to have a negative article published about something the administration was behind. *(Sheila Burke was a staff member in Mike Bisciglia's office who was responsible for press releases and community relations)*.

1/29–I spoke with an administrator at NYCC who informed me that NYCC's accreditation with the CCE had been re-affirmed for a period of two years. There seems to be a significant amount of animosity between the administration and the faculty union here at UB. Several news articles have appeared in the *Telegram*, a local newspaper highlighting the conflict.

In addition to the financial problems faced by the university, the hostility between the administration and faculty was another item which should have been shared with me before I became involved in the project.

(The animosity between the administration and faculty on campus was palpable. While originally I was confused as to why faculty ignored me, I soon understood I was seen as an agent of the administration—I was the enemy.)

1/30–Dinner meeting with Arnold, Bob, Marc Peyser, Janet Greenwood *(president of the university)*, Ed Eigel and George Mihalakos *(university attorney)*, wherein the university agreed on the role of the Steering Committee, so now we can start fundraising in earnest. Ed Eigel returned the licensure application. It needs a few minor edits. The edits will be made, the application re-submitted to him one more time, then off to the state.

1/31–I worked all morning on the licensure application. I want to get it to Ed Eigel by Friday. If I get it back on Monday I can send it out to be bound and mail it to the state.

In the meantime I have a list of assignments which emerged from the dinner meeting the other night. Now it's just a matter of getting the job done.

(*In January 1990 the first program update was submitted to the Chiropractic College Committee. The topics addressed were the number of student inquiries (61) which were received from the tristate area and California, Wisconsin, Vermont, Rhode Island, Massachusetts and Georgia. Twenty-six prospective faculty from around the country also contacted the university to inquire about the program. The Council on Chiropractic Education was contacted for the first time in January 1990.[3] The encouraging information in the update was the diversity of student and faculty inquiries. When at NYCC, student inquiries were routinely confined to the tristate area. Faculty inquiries came from across the country. Obviously, the lure of university employment appealed to individuals willing to teach in the chiropractic program*).

2/2–One of the dinner meeting assignments I was given was to develop letters to be sent to prospective faculty and students. I sent Dr. Eigel completed versions of the letters as well as the revised, completed licensure application.

I received a call from Dr. Eigel asking whether or not he should meet with Keith Overland, the president of the Connecticut Chiropractic Association. I called Marc Peyser to inquire about the meeting request and he indicated it was legitimate. Marc thought it would be okay for the provost to meet with Keith as long as I was there because Keith has a habit of running off at the mouth. An hour later Marc called to advise me he would have the meeting with Keith. I stated this was a good idea because the last thing we need is for chiropractors to start calling and taking up Eigel's time. Marc said all calls from the profession should be forwarded to the members of the Steering Committee.

2/5–I was informed that Dominic Fiorillo, PhD, was offered the academic VP position at NYCC. I received the contact letters back from Dr. Eigel today. I think the reason I got them today was because I delivered the names and addresses of the Steering Committee to his secretary. In addition I picked up the tape of the news show from Sheila Burke and made arrangements for our rebuttal to the AAUP newsletter to be printed in a special edition of the *Bulletin*–the weekly publication of UB.

More calls from prospective students. I made a lunch date to meet with Rose Galiger, the pre-chiro advisor here at UB. I will have lunch with her next Monday.

(*My first meeting with Dr. Galiger was similar to every other meeting which had happened between myself and other faculty—it was adversarial. Dr. Galiger expressed anger at being involved in the pre-chiropractic program at UB and had not been extended the courtesy of being asked her opinion about the proposed chiropractic program*).

2/7–Busy day. Sent out letters to prospective students and faculty. Received inquiries from five more students. Received a packet of information from L.F. O'Connell (PR Firm) and another from the CCE. We should get the accreditation process started soon.

2/9–I sent out a few more letters to prospective students. Since I picked up a hole-puncher and binders I started putting the licensure document together. Now all I need is the document which Ed Eigel has. Once I receive his material, the books can be out of my office in a matter of hours.

Called NYCC—everybody in meetings. I wonder what's going on? Unofficial enrollment projections for April 1990 indicate the class size to be in the twenties. Usually the actual number falls short of the projected number. Just what NYCC needs, another class that starts with fewer students than anticipated. That will not help their financial picture.

(*Fortunately Dr. Napolitano left NYCC with a huge endowment. His frugality and securing Bundy Aid helped to build the endowment which would help stabilize their financial posture for years to come.*)

Finished the week with 76 student inquiries and 37 faculty inquiries. I would like to get 100 student inquiries by 3/15/90. This number is doable.

2/12–Picked up a lot of office supplies on Saturday and packed them away this morning. Ed Eigel called, the report is finished. All I need to do is type up his part and run off the necessary copies.

2/15–Applications for licensure were submitted to Ed Eigel who said they could be sent out tomorrow. I turned $19,300 in checks over to Mike Bisciglia's office. Met with Marc Dionne of L. F. O'Connell regarding a PR piece which will be mailed out by August 1990. Picked up two more prospective students, now at 82. Now I can discuss specific aspects of the program since the licensure application is completed.

2/16–Finished collating licensure application. Had lunch with Sheila Burke who told me about yesterday's Trustees meeting. Dr. Eigel reported to the board the licensure application for the chiropractic program has been sent to the state.

Received faculty and student transcripts which I started filing. I also made up files for administrative personnel and special events.

Joan from Dr. Eigel's office called to ask how to handle a call from a Dr. Bazakos. I called Bob to ask him how the call should be handled and he told me to find out what's going on. I called Dr. Bazakos a couple of times and the call did not go through. When my call finally did connect, he was at lunch. I tried several more times to reach Dr. Bazakos, each time he was busy.

Spoke with Bob Matrisciano and he told me Val Pasqua had gotten in touch with Bud Passero stating there should be no "bad blood" between the schools and suggested UB might want to send a representative to Dr. Ken Padgett's investiture. Bud responded he was not involved in the Bridgeport project, but in his opinion, Bob Matrisciano would be a good representative of the program. At this point Pasqua indicated he would have to get back to Bud. I think these guys in New York may be 1.) trying to get Bud involved and 2.) are very concerned about the progress we are making. I think part of the reaction is because we have sent letters to prospective students and faculty advising them to send transcripts to the university. This information had to get back to the powers that be.

(*Val Pasqua, D.C. was a member of the "old guard" who had been ousted from power when Bob Matrisciano was elected president of NYSCA. Dr. Pasqua's call seeking peace between the programs was strange. There was no program at the University of Bridgeport at this time. Ken Padgett, D.C., formerly a member of the NYCC Board of Trustees had been elected president of the college, replacing Keith Asplin, PhD*)

2/19–As yet, Dr. Bazakos has not gotten in touch with me. It's funny, for a guy who has been trying diligently to contact Dr. Eigel, he has found precious little time to talk to me. I guess he needed to find out what to say to me. Today is President's Day which means most of the world is closed (i.e., Postal Service), however I have been able to keep busy with other things in the office. Life goes on.

2/21–Got letters out to more prospective students and faculty. Called Marc Peyser to ask whether or not I should respond to the CCA's request to write a letter in support of a bill to allow chiropractors to perform sports physicals.

Started to prepare my monthly report to the Steering Committee. To date I have not heard about the Steering Committee Bylaws revisions which were supposed to be completed by George Mihalakos. Still no word on the fundraising brochure.

2/23–Got licensure application out to the Steering Committee as well as other correspondence. Spoke with George Mihalakos who indicated the bylaws have been completed. After review by the president they will be forwarded to me for distribution to the committee members. Sent out program update to Steering Committee; 88 students and 40 faculty.

2/26–Met for over an hour with Dean Nechascek. We talked about the program, the role of the university faculty, anatomy labs and licensing. Dean Nechascek thought our program would get state approval, but he also indicated the university will be in for some serious turmoil in the next few months wherein many members of the current administration are in jeopardy of losing their jobs.

A few more student inquiries today, although mail has been slow.

2/28–Received more transcripts from prospective students and faculty. Received transfer directory from Jackie Benamati asking if we wanted to get involved in the project. I will need to review the book and get back to her.

(*Two program updates were submitted in February 1990. The number of student inquiries increased to 88. The number of faculty inquiries increased to 40. The home locations of inquiries increased to include: Vermont, New Hampshire, Maine, Pennsylvania and Virginia. The licensure application was submitted to the state*).[4]

3/2–As soon as I got in the office I received a call from Joe Nechasek who said he had spoken to a student at NYCC who told him many students are looking to transfer out of NYCC to other schools. We then spoke about what I thought might be happening at NYCC.

Last Wednesday, a Westchester chiropractor made a similar inquiry asking if the chiropractic program at UB would be accepting transfer students.

Spoke with Dr. Miller of the Faculty Council and Chemistry Department. He and his colleagues are QUITE upset about how the university went about establishing a chiropractic program without their input. I told Dr. Miller I was unable to speak to the process, but was more than willing to meet with members of the faculty to discuss the chiropractic program. Dr. Miller felt it was too late because the licensure application had already been submitted. I reiterated my offer to meet with the faculty council and explain the chiropractic program to them. I indicated Dr. Miller should send me a calendar of when the meetings are held and I would be happy to attend.

I went to have lunch with Dr. Singletary (Biology) who forgot and wasn't there. I called him at three o'clock at which time he apologized profusely. We made another appointment.

I met with Gus Seaman *(Head of Purchasing)* who showed me the offices in the nursing building. They are all small. I chose room 220. I will inform Catherine Yang as soon as possible.

Joan from Dr. Eigel's office called to assure me the licensure application went out on 2/14/90. This is the wrap-up to the Miller phone call earlier today.

I called NYCC to speak with Dr. Padgett, but he was not there. I then spoke with John Pecchia *(NYCC VP of Finance)* to tell him what I had heard about NYCC students looking to transfer. I advised John I would call Ken back next week.

(Faculty at the University of Bridgeport had an inflated opinion of the importance of their input into the planning process. While their technical expertise could be helpful, their inability to see the big picture was a fatal flaw. With the licensure application in process, and after reading why the university should not start a chiropractic program in the AAUP newsletter, I thought it would be beneficial if I met with the senior members of the

basic science faculty. I met with representatives from Biology, Chemistry and Physics. I could tell by their body language they were not interested in wasting their time in a meeting with a chiropractor.)

I introduced myself and explained my role at the University

"What is your educational background?"

"I have a B.S. in Psychology from St. Peter's College and a D.C. from the New York Chiropractic College."

The first order of business was to have these PhDs explain to me that a clinical degree such as a D.C. in an academic environment meant nothing. The only degree of value was an academic degree (PhD or EdD) To ensure I understood and was not offended, my academic colleagues assured me the rules were for all clinical degrees, including an M.D., D.O., or D.D.S.

After I thanked them for explaining the hierarchy of academia to me I stated my reason for inviting them to this meeting. I had spoken to several members of the faculty who expressed various degrees of negative emotions at the manner in which the chiropractic project was begun and had proceeded, and I wanted to answer any questions they might have.

"What kind of experience do you have in administration?"

I proceeded to tell them about my positions at NYCC and my experience with accreditation when I was again interrupted, "So you have no experience in higher education?"

"Well, the New York Chiropractic College—"

"Is a chiropractic school. That hardly qualifies as higher education. An individual can be admitted to a chiropractic school even if they do not graduate from high school."

Another added, "A chiropractic school is really a technical school, without the academic rigors of an accredited institution of higher learning. You realize the University of Bridgeport is accredited by the New England Association of Schools and Colleges, in addition to the individual programs within the university being accredited by specialized agencies, such as the engineering school and the law school."

I could feel the anger rising up inside of me, but I was able to maintain my composure.

"So the fact of the matter is, you are attempting to start this chiropractic program here at the University of Bridgeport and it clearly does not have the pedigree or quality to be part of the university's current offerings. Why should we support this undertaking?"

I finally had the opportunity to speak. "Because I'm going to make you money."

The people sitting around the table were shocked. "Money?"

"That's what you people need. You need money and I need a home. Now if you don't want the money my program can bring into the university, fine. I'll take the program someplace else."

I had nowhere else to go, but these pompous asses didn't know that. The only thing they knew was they were PhDs and they were at the top of the food chain in their environment.

I continued, "You boys are spoiled. You are in the habit of getting paid regularly because state or federal funds balance your budget. That's no longer the case. Look around you at what's happening here at UB. You're going broke, and the cavalry is not coming to the rescue. The College of Chiropractic is." The room was filled with myself and six other people, there were no sounds, not even breathing.

"Now are you ready to learn about chiropractic education and the plans for this project, or is this meeting over?"

I then proceeded to explain how the College of Chiropractic would be a great addition to the university. I spoke about the courses in the curriculum and the process of professional accreditation which we would need to achieve to qualify our students for licensure, as well as the prerequisites for admission. The College of Chiropractic was not a technical school. The admission requirements were the same, in terms of course work, as the requirements to be accepted into medical school.

(By the time the meeting was over, two points were clear. The senior members of the basic science faculty knew factually what chiropractic education was, and appeared to be favorably impressed and these same individuals did not like the director of the chiropractic program.)

3/5–called NYCC, advised Dr. Padgett was at upstate campus; left message I would call back on Wednesday morning.

Designed application form, picked up two more prospective student inquiries. Visited Lucy Marini in graduate admissions and received the names of two financial aid people who work with graduate students. Have a meeting on Friday with Bessie Phakias *(Financial Aid)*.

Spoke with Arnold and Bob, things pretty much status quo. Bob had a meeting with Mollie Donovan *(longtime assistant to Ernest Napolitano, president of Columbia Institute of Chiropractic and NYCC)* on Thursday.

Received a call from the President of the Faculty Council requesting a meeting with me next week. It appears the administration and faculty have an extremely adversarial relationship.

3/7–Started the accreditation process by copying a list of the information we need to submit to the Council on Chiropractic Education (CCE). I will meet with Ed Eigel to get the documents we need from his office. I hope to submit this information to the CCE by May 1, 1990.

Gave Arnold the fax number so that he could have Bud fax a copy of the brochure so that I can fax it back after reviewing and we can get the brochure OUT!!!

(The fundraising efforts of the Chiropractic College Committee had still not started. The initial effort was supposed to begin in October 1989, with a follow up initiative to begin in January 1990. The rationale for these efforts not starting was the lack of a written agreement between the Committee and UB. Next, the lack of a fundraising brochure stood in the way of the committee members soliciting funds.

The money which had sustained the project so far has been primarily raised by Dr. Matrisciano.)

3/9–Met with Bessie Phakias and Norma Abrams-McNerney of UB Financial Aid this morning. Picked up a couple more students and faculty today, more transcripts have come in.

Went to look at my new office, room 220 in the nursing building. I will be moving there next week. Mailed out a report to the Steering Committee. I have yet to receive a finalized version of the agreement between the university and us (Chiropractic College Committee).

Japanese contingent on campus. The talk around campus is that these individuals will be purchasing some acreage and buildings for $18 million.

Ken Padgett never called me back. I guess chiropractors in New York are all too busy to return phone calls.

3/12–Spoke with Lou Sportelli regarding the brochure which finally seems to be getting started. Lou anticipates completion by the end of the month. I spoke with Arnold who feels the timing for the brochure is bad and it will be very difficult to raise the $500,000 needed by the end of June. Arnold indicated the brochure should have been completed a couple of months ago. When I was complaining about the lack of planning on the brochure, I was told there were other things going on. Now as it is obvious we are up against the wall, now he feels the planning should have been better coordinated.

(Louis Sportelli, D.C., is a prominent chiropractic activist who has become a spokesperson for the chiropractic profession due to his eloquence. He has also authored a variety of publications in addition to being involved in state, national and international politics. Dr. Sportelli had been contacted by Dr. Cianciulli, his close personal friend, to have his company produce the fundraising brochure).[5]

Had lunch with Dr. Singletary who was basically supportive but non-committal about the project. He then told me about the history of UB. He has been at UB for 19 years. Today the university is announcing a restructuring plan that will affect all employees. This is a way to cut some of the excess fat out of the faculty, by firing people who are not carrying their weight. Needless to say, Dr. Singletary is concerned about his job and the jobs of fellow faculty members.

(The University of Bridgeport was in serious financial trouble at this time, largely because common sense, in an environment of learned people, did not exist. For instance, the student enrollment at UB peaked in 1979 at slightly less than 10,000 students. When I arrived in 1989, enrollment was approximately 5,000 students. Unfortunately, the administrative structure which had supported 10,000 students was exactly the same—supporting 5,000. While revenue had been decreased by 50%, expenses remained the same.

My first week at UB I was walking down the hall in the Dana Building where a class was being conducted by a tenured faculty member to four students. I went to the registrar's office and asked the registrar, "Was that a special class I just saw?"

"No, it was a regular class."

"Don't you have a minimum number of students who must register for a class in order for that class to be run by the university?"

"We do, but we don't."

"Could you explain the policy?"

"There are supposed to be at least 15 people registered for a class to run. If there are less than that, the dean has the authority to contact the registrar and permit the class to be held."

"How can UB hold classes where the faculty member's salary was not being covered by the tuition paid by the students?"

"We do it all the time," was the answer.

Lack of common sense and poor business practices were the recipe for disaster which had brought UB to this point. The financial crisis the university was experiencing threatened the existence of the institution. It also threatened to rob the university of its future—the College of Chiropractic.

In the back of my head were the words Dr. Napolitano had shared with me when I told him I wanted to become involved in chiropractic education. "Remember, it's a business. If you don't make more than you spend, you can't remain in business. Never forget, it's a business." Certainly, based upon his experience, Dr. Napolitano knew the challenges of running an academic institution. Chiropractic education was not the beneficiary of state or federal funding. It was not the beneficiary of philanthropic gifts. It functioned on the basis of modest tuition revenue and frugal business practices.)

Spoke with Bob and he indicated he backed off asking Mollie Donovan for money, but he will pursue this at another time.

Good day for student calls. If we keep this up, we will have 200 prospective students by May!

3/14–Mailed letters out and received more transcripts. Received a call from another NYCC student who stated morale is low and half the student body is on probation, and a good number of students are looking to transfer out. I called a friend at the NYCC registrar's office who basically confirmed the morale issue, but emphatically stated there was no mass exodus occurring at the school. She indicated, according to her records, total enrollment was 670 students.

3/16–I arrived on campus this morning to find out I am not moving into the nursing building. Instead I am being relocated to room 246 in Rennell Hall. This is not a big deal. As a matter of fact it might be better to reside in a building surrounded by a lot of people (and information) as opposed to being in a building where there is never anyone around. The move took up the entire day. However, by the time I left Friday night I was settled in and ready to go. I met Bob Green, the UB bursar who appears to be a nice guy who "tells it like it is." The rest of the staff in the building seem very nice.

3/19–Met with Margot Hardenberg (*President of the Faculty Council*) this morning. She asked me about the program, duration, prerequisites, etc. and then expressed some concern over the lack of faculty input into the program. I told her our program is in the planning phase and will evolve into a mature program. As a result I told her not to compare our program to other university programs that have already matured. I told her I appreciated her concerns and at the appropriate time any problematic areas she or other members of the faculty council identify will be addressed. I also indicated anyone on the faculty who does not support the philosophy of chiropractic will not be invited to be part of our faculty. The meeting lasted an hour, was cordial and I indicated if Margot needed additional information , or if she felt it was important for me to speak with a particular individual, she should simply call upon me.

I made an appointment with George Mihalakos on Wednesday to pick up accreditation material I will need for the CCE.

3/24–Met with George Mihalakos and briefed him on the information I will need for the eligibility document. He also indicated the Steering Committee guidelines are being completed and will be sent to me as soon as they are finished. Hopefully, it will not be too long.

I asked Lillian Nash to record the outgoing message on our answering machine. She did a good job. Now all we need is to have the phone turned on. We have been without the use of a phone for three and one half days—this situation is killing us. God knows how many calls we have lost and what kind of thoughts are going through the minds of people trying to reach us.

3/23–After calling the office several times yesterday I came to the realization the phone was not connected properly. Instead of hooking it up to 576-4279, it was hooked up to 576-4297. The problem was rectified this morning.

I ordered new business cards today. The ones I had for Halsey Hall had chiropractic misspelled on them anyway. I hope I can have these new cards in about two weeks. In the meantime, I will continue to use what I have.

I received several calls from prospective students today, all of whom have been trying to reach me for a week. In an hour I picked up three more prospective applicants.

George Mihalakos came by the office and asked for a concise outline of the CCE Standards so the Board of Trustees will be able to vote on a resolution to adopt the standards as required by the CCE for eligibility.

Received the financial audit dated December 31, 1989.

3/26–Interviewed a prospective student today. Processed mail. This week has already been the most student inquiries received. I would like to be up to 140 inquiries by the time I submit my next report to the Steering Committee. George Mihalakos gave me the completed Steering Committee guidelines on Friday which I mailed to the members via registered mail on Saturday.[6]

Met with prospective student referred by a NJ chiropractor.

Spoke with Ralph Miller today regarding when to submit our eligibility document. Ralph suggested we wait until November/December 1991. This will be two years after we started compliance with CCE admissions criteria.

3/30–Slow, aggravating day. I got in the office to find the answering machine is broken. The information needed for the brochure has not been received by Sheila Burke. No mail, minimal phone calls. I met with a Connecticut D.C. who is looking to become a faculty member at UB. Other than that, the day has been like the weather, dark, rainy, sucky.

(March program updates indicated an increase in student inquiries to 115. Faculty transcripts have been arriving and now number 22. Work continued on the CCE eligibility document. I reported my initial meeting with the President of the Faculty Council and announced the move of my office from Halsey Hall to Rennell Hall. The Advisory Council guidelines were received from George Mihalakos and submitted to the Advisory Council for their review and approval). [7]

4/2–Another slow day. For the first time in a long time no student inquiries. A couple of phone calls, but nothing significant, Ed Eigel called to tell me the president wants a weekly report on progress. I spoke with Keith Overland and I will be speaking before the Connecticut Chiropractic Association on Thursday evening. Other than that all is very quiet.

4/4–Slow, quiet day. Nothing significant seems to be happening anywhere.

4/5–Spoke before the CCA in Waterbury. Contrary to what I have been told by Keith, there appears to be a strong, vocal, negative sentiment expressed by the CCA membership about the Bridgeport project. On a positive note, speaking one-on-one to members in the audience, support was voiced for our efforts. Janet Greenwood made a nice presentation and I met Sara Melendez for the first time. She is the assistant provost. A CCA member pledged $10,000 to the effort. He did so in front of the membership. (Pledge was never honored).

(The biggest objection voiced by members of the CCA about the college being in Connecticut was the state would be saturated with chiropractors just like every state that houses a chiropractic program. There were no questions or comments from the membership about what benefits the program could mean to each of them individually or the CCA in general. The only question I was asked was where I was from. When I responded New York, the majority of the audience lost interest in the presentation. I learned quickly if you wanted to do business in Connecticut, it was best to be from Connecticut.)

4/6–Called Fred Bass from Lippincott Books to thank him for the books he sent and to make an appointment for us to review the curriculum and see what additional books he may have for the program. Fred called back and we set a date for 4/27/90.

Got a call from Lou Sportelli's office regarding the brochure. Janet Greenwood made some last minute changes. The brochure should be completed next week.

Spoke with Bob Matrisciano and he informed me that two NYCC principals would be opening a restaurant and hotel in upstate New York. Bob doing homework on a convention. Federation of Chiropractic Societies will be conducting a continuing education seminar sponsored by Parker College of Chiropractic. Proceeds would be donated to support our efforts at UB. (The seminar was never held.)

(Dr. Alessandro Pireno, a longtime friend and supporter of Dr. Matrisciano, *was a principal in the Federated Societies organization. His support of the Bridgeport initiative was based solely on Dr. Matrisciano's involvement in the project. As committed as Dr. Pireno was to Dr. Matrisciano, he was equally adversarial to Dr. Cianciulli, which meant money might come from New York, through Alex, but it would not flow easily or fast).*

4/9–Attended NYCC's graduation yesterday. Students and graduates to whom I spoke were very appreciative of my attending the ceremony and excited about our efforts at UB. The ceremony itself was not one of the best. The microphone did not work properly, Frank DeGiacomo was the Grand Marshall, the commencement address was radical and the procession disorganized. The welcome to the profession speech, delivered by college Trustee Edward Epstein, D.C., who called Dr. Padgett NYCC's new father and NYCC has two new uncles in Dr. Fiorello and Dr. Faust. Talk about a dysfunctional family. Arno Burnier, D.C., challenged the graduates to forget what they learned in school and adjust subluxations. The people on stage looked somewhat uncomfortable at his statements. All in all I think it was a day that most people at NYCC would like to forget.

In general, a quiet day at the university. I did hear some interesting information though. It seems two senior NYCC faculty members, Frank Langilotti and Frank Giacomo are looking to move Alan Friedman, D.C., the current director of the Levittown clinic out as director when NYCC moves upstate. The rationale is plain and simple, they will then have jobs downstate and not have to move. I also heard from John Bonsignor yesterday that he is being phased out of his job of going to conventions by Mark Feldman, D.C., who was assigned my responsibilities when I left NYCC. Another casualty is Mike Bruzik who will be leaving NYCC at the end of summer.

(The responsibilities of the Division of Student Affairs included Public Relations and Alumni Affairs. John Bonsignor was an asset in the area of PR. He hosted a local radio show on Sundays and knew many local business owners. Mike Bruzik was instrumental in developing Chiropractic Today, a cable television program which was instrumental in helping to teach viewers the various aspects of chiropractic care. The consensus of people was that chiropractors "crack people's backs." Chiropractic Today was an award winning

cable television program.)

Went through inquiries today. 50% male, 50% female. Aside from that, no news because there was no mail delivery.

4/13–Things continue to be quiet. The mail is not coming in until late in the day, so today I opened Monday and Tuesday's mail. I have no intention of staying all day Friday so I guess mail is going to be a problem.

Spent part of the day studying for my court appearance. I will meet with John Henry tomorrow to review the case. (*I was an expert witness in a malpractice case.*)

Hopefully, the brochures are being run and money will be coming into the system soon. I am supposed to speak before a group of Suffolk County (New York) chiropractors tomorrow evening. I need to get the relevant information from Bob.

4/15–Spoke to the Suffolk County chiropractors last night. A small group but very emotional and confused about the state of chiropractic politics in New York. Got in to school to find the university closed. Copied my phone messages, made entry in diary, made some calls and headed back to New York.

4/16–I called Ed Eigel to inquire about the status of our licensure application and he advised me of the following: 1) the investigator has been changed from Lisa Stamons to John Walters; 2) there is a question regarding our funding; 3) there is a regulation of the state which mandates a doctor's degree can be given three years after completion of a baccalaureate degree. We will need to see the specific wording of the regulation before we proceed. Ed Eigel feels the next step is a meeting with the state to discuss these issues. In the meantime, I need to get hold of the state regulations which are being quoted.

(*A meeting was eventually held in December between myself and Norma Glasgow, the Commissioner of Education and her staff. At that meeting it was explained the state regulation called for a doctoral degree to be conferred seven years after achieving a secondary diploma. The interpretation of this regulation, by the staff of the Department of Higher Education, was four years after achieving a secondary diploma, a baccalaureate degree would be achieved. After achieving a baccalaureate degree, a doctoral degree could be achieved. The DHE staff indicated to get into medical school a baccalaureate degree is required, therefore a baccalaureate degree should be the requirement for chiropractic school.*

The prerequisites to enter chiropractic school, at that time, was a minimum of 60 undergraduate credits to include courses in biology, chemistry, organic chemistry and physics, as well as psychology, arts, and humanities. This meant a chiropractic candidate could attend two years undergraduate training, before entering a ten-trimester professional program. Ten trimesters, a year-round program, divided by two (Fall and Spring), a traditional academic year, equals five years. Two undergraduate years plus five years of professional (chiropractic) school equals seven years of study past a secondary diploma. The minimum requirements for medical school were 90 undergraduate credits, prior to four years of medical school. Three years of undergraduate school, plus four years of medical school equals seven.

According to my research and analysis both programs met the requirements of the state regulations. Commissioner Glasgow agreed with my analysis. She did however partially side with her staff. The meeting ended with my agreeing to require a chiropractic candidate attend a minimum of three years undergraduate school before being eligible to attend the chiropractic program at the University of Bridgeport. Eventually, the Council on Chiropractic Education adopted three years of undergraduate training as a prerequisite for all accredited chiropractic programs, years after the prerequisite was adopted at the University of Bridgeport. One institution had to be first, in this case it would UBCC, and we were not yet licensed.

At the time of this issue, I thoroughly reviewed the admission requirements of medical schools in the United States. Of the 125 medical schools in the United States, seven required a baccalaureate degree for admission. These programs were:

University of Illinois   University of Minnesota (Duluth)
Loyola University of Chicago University of Minnesota (Minneapolis)
Mayo Medical College   Ohio State University
Uniformed Services University of the Health Sciences

Neither of the two medical programs in the state of Connecticut, Yale or the University of Connecticut, was on the list of schools which required a baccalaureate degree. This fact supported my contention that the State Department of Education was imposing a higher standard of admission on UB's chiropractic program than was expected of medical programs.)[8]

Aside from that, Jean Southard informed me the check for Unigraphic was ready to be mailed. There were two more potential students from Massachusetts.

(*Unigraphic was the company producing the fundraising brochures. A year after negotiations had been initiated with representatives of the chiropractic profession and the University of Bridgeport a fundraising brochure was finally going out in the mail to solicit funds*).

4/18–Slow phone day, but several student inquiries from Texas. Still no word from the state regarding specific questions with the licensure application.

Tomorrow I will speak to a group of chiropractors at the Carlen Hotel, courtesy of the Federation of Chiropractic Societies.

The fundraising brochure was to have been mailed out yesterday. Hopefully money should start coming into the program.

I wonder if it might not be advantageous to run a piece in *Dynamic Chiropractic*?

4/20–Since this journal began we have averaged 6.24 student inquiries a week. Since 1/16/90 we have averaged 7.38 student inquiries per week. So far the best month we have had is March with 45 inquiries. April should break 30 with little trouble. Surprisingly the inquiries from Massachusetts and Rhode Island have been strong with Massachusetts rivalling New Jersey.

To date, based on total inquiries, the percentage from each state is:

State	Total Number of Inquiries	Percentage of Total Inquiries
Connecticut	63	40
New York	35	22
New Jersey	18	12
Massachusetts	18	12
Rhode Island	5	3
Texas	3	2
California	3	2
New Hampshire	2	<1%
Maine	2	<1%
Vermont	1	<1%
Virginia	2	<1%
Pennsylvania	1	<1%
Iowa	1	<1%
Wisconsin	1	<1%

(The inaugural UBCC graduating class consisted of students from Connecticut, New Jersey and Massachusetts.)

Even though activity has been slow this week, I anticipate it picking up next week after the fundraising brochure is mailed out.

I just got off the phone with Lou Sportelli's office. The fundraising brochure should be out by Wednesday of next week. Hopefully an article will appear in *Dynamic Chiropractic* to coincide with this momentous event.

4/23–Received a call from Lou Sportelli who was wondering where the check for the brochures is? I went to see Jean Southard who informed me the check is scheduled to be mailed on 4/26/90. I called Lou back to inform him and he was not too pleased. He then told me how much the postage was going to cost and I wrote out a requisition and sent it to Mike Bisciglia. My initial requisition for the fundraising brochure went to Mike Bisciglia on 4/9. Over two weeks before a check can be mailed? The bureaucracy in this place is stifling!

Aside from receiving a call from Lou Sportelli the day has been exceptionally dead. With the exception of a meeting on Friday with Fred Bass from Lippincott I don't know how much more will be happening until additional money is deposited in the treasury. With the requisition of postage, the cost of brochures and my salary, we have spent almost $30,000—which means we are almost broke.

4/25–Received a call from a 2nd tri student at NYCC who indicated a significant number of students would be willing to transfer if the accreditation issues can be adequately addressed. Picked up another student today. It would be nice to have 200 by June 1, 1990. Aside from that all else is quiet.

On Friday I will start pressing for answers to the state position on our licensure.

It's amazing, but most people work at such a low level of efficiency that a minimal amount of work will keep them busy a maximum amount of time. I wonder what it would be like to live on a farm, in a small house, a thousand miles away from this insanity. This is something I would like to experience.

4/27–Met with Fred Bass today. He will be sending me a couple more books for possible use in the program. I had the pleasure of talking with Arnold who informed me we were down to our last $1200 and we need to get more money into the till. The project is going to go, but we need the green!

Picked up some more prospective students—the number is now 163. This for a class of 65.

4/30–Day started off with my getting a memo and check for $2500 to Mike Bisciglia. Spoke with Arnold and informed him I would be meeting with NYCC students at my home in Long Island about the possibility of transferring. I also spoke to him about the fundraising brochure which is still being held up pending receipt of a check.

I met Ed Eigel in the hall and he said he still hasn't heard anything from the state yet. If he still hasn't heard anything by the end of the week he will call them and check on the status.

I found out from Jean Southard the check for the fundraising brochures was not mailed out last week but would be mailed out today. I told her not to mail it and Federal Expressed it through Mike Beecher's office. *(Vice President of Finance)* Lillian Nash, as usual, helped me get it out. I spoke with Marc Peyser and Bud about the brochure and they seemed disappointed. I reminded them they are dealing with a complex bureaucracy.

At least now I know the check has been mailed. I also processed the invoice for Maxwell Peterson Publishing for the labels for the brochures. The balance of the money on hand should last for two weeks.

(The April program update indicated 148 student inquiries and 53 faculty inquiries. The Advisory Council was apprised, for the first time, of the amount of money which had been received to support the project. The number of student and faculty inquiries continued to grow on a regular basis, fundraising continued to be dismal). [9]

5/2–Picked up seven prospective students today. Calculated the cost of the program by credit and by the hour. Spoke with Lou Sportelli who informed me the brochures went out yesterday with advance copies going to the appropriate individuals. Got a call from President Greenwood checking on the status of the brochures and finances. In two weeks the new Trustees will be announced and she was hoping Bob Matrisciano would be placed on the board at that time for political reasons. I spoke with Bob and it looks like his appointment will have to wait because the chances of us making half a million dollars in two weeks is negligible. Aside from that—all quiet on the western front.

(The fundraising brochures were finally mailed on May 1, 1990! They should have been prepared and mailed seven months ago. The system to follow-up on the brochures should have been designed and implemented seven months ago. For all intents and purposes, the project should be starting now. It appears now is too late.)

5/4–Got in the office this morning to find a case of brochures. Finally, the finished product! Picked up several more prospective students. The number is now 176.

I spoke again with Janet Greenwood who indicated she would be willing to put Bob on the Trustees if the response we are getting from the brochure makes it look like we are going to make the half million dollars by the end of June 1990. Got paid again today. Ken Padgett's investiture is tomorrow and I will be in attendance. Spoke with Walt

Wardwell (chiropractic historian) and we will have lunch together next Wednesday at UConn.

The brochures for the Genesis Fund were professionally produced and looked great! There were eight sections to the brochure. The first was a picture of Janet Greenwood along with a letter describing the university and how the College of Chiropractic will benefit the profession. The brochure opens to an aerial view of the university and a description of the goals of the project.

Opening the brochure there are two testimonials by an orthopedic surgeon and radiologist, in addition to a panel which has facts about the university (enrollment 5300). The next panel are pictures of the individuals on the Genesis Committee:

A.E.Cianciulli–New Jersey   R.D. Mastronardi–Rhode Island
M. Peyser–ConnecticutP.   P.H. Bosen–New Hampshire
R. Matrisciano–New York   J. Danchik–Massachusetts
J. Gnall–Pennsylvania   R. Lynch–Maine

The final panel was a letter from the program director with a pledge card on the opposite side. There was an envelope with the brochure addressed to Genesis Fund, c/o VP Michael Bisciglia–University of Bridgeport.

5/7–Went to Ken Padgett's investiture on Saturday. Most chiropractic colleges had someone in attendance. Presidents included Bea Hagen (Logan) Sid Williams (Life) Gerry Clum (Life-West) John Miller (Palmer West) and Matthew Givrard (CEO elect LACC). The other schools sent representatives, except Parker, Texas and Western States.

Several more student inquiries. I sent some brochures to Mike Bisciglia's office.

5/9–Aggravating day. I tried to meet with Walt Wardwell and got stuck on I95—both ways! Missed the appointment and spent about six hours on the road, in addition to the other hours I usually spend traveling. Other than that, all is quiet.

5/11–The brochures seem to be making a small impact. Ken Padgett told Beth Donohue I have "balls bigger than an elephant." He also believes we will never raise the money. The first call I received today was a pledge of $1,000 from a chiropractor in Randolph, Massachusetts.

Spoke with Arnold who said the phone chain will be up and running next week. He told me to get some PR information to *Dynamic Chiropractic*. He also told me to call a member of the committee from New Hampshire. I called—this guy sounds like a real prize—he got a brochure the other day, but didn't know what it was about.

(*The individual's picture was on the brochure and he was supposed to be one of the people soliciting money for the project! It became obvious to me that the individuals on the committee were asked to have their pictures placed on the brochure, but not to actively participate in raising funds. The individuals who were supposed to be raising money had no idea of the enormity of the assignment. They were not fundraisers, but chiropractic politicians.*)

The fundraising aspect of this initiative is the weakest link for a variety of reasons. One, it is difficult to get people to donate money. Two, the coordination and communication between the Steering Committee members has been poor. In fact, with the exception of Bob Matrisciano, there is a definite reluctance to get the job done. This has been apparent from day one. The fact that it took over three months to produce and distribute a fundraising brochure has weakened our credibility. There have been no articles in the chiropractic journals or newspapers. Most people who know what is going on have found out by word of mouth, from people on the periphery of the project.

The road blocks we faced seemed not too critical, but they now loom larger than ever. First we were reluctant to pursue fundraising because the bylaws regarding the Steering Committee were questionable. That issue was addressed. Then, we couldn't get the brochures printed because the company printing the brochures was committed to other assignments. When the company was finally available, the money to pay for the job was not mailed out in a timely fashion and an additional week was tacked on the wait.

When I originally got involved in this project I was told money would not be a problem. The math was simple. "All we need is 1,000 chiropractors to donate $1,000," and we would have all the money necessary. I was also told there was a fund controlled by UB board member and chiropractic supporter Carmen Tortora which would be used to finance the venture. I was also told that there was a Connecticut D.C. who had a family business who would donate big bucks to the venture if the D.C. would be named to the Steering Committee. I have no doubt there is money out there. I just don't think there is an organized, serious effort to secure these funds.

5/14–Got a call from Lou Sportelli inquiring about the $2171.00 needed to pay for the postage on the brochures. After checking, I advised him the money would be mailed on Friday, at which time I was advised that the next time Unigraphics does anything with UB payment will be in hand first. I went to lunch with Walter Feller who agreed to teach Jurisprudence for no salary. He also offered to perform any additional legal help we might need pro bono. He also talked about NYCC. He indicated Tony Onorato was having a difficult time deciding whether or not he should make the move to Seneca Falls.

I called Ed Eigel who indicated the state is still fiddling around with the licensure application. For the first time in a long time, there were no calls from prospective students today. Do they know something I don't?

(Anthony Onorato, D.C., was originally hired by me as an adjunct faculty member at NYCC. Because of his performance in the classroom and clinic he was promoted to Director of Clinical Sciences before assuming the position of Director of Clinical and Chiropractic Sciences. Due to the instability and volatility at NYCC, he was named Acting Vice President of Academic Affairs. With the appointment of Dominic Fiorillo as Vice President of Academic Affairs, Dr. Onorato assumed the position of Dean of Academic Affairs. He did move to Seneca Falls briefly when the college relocated to upstate New York. His home and family were based in downstate New York, and the lack of leadership and focus at the new NYCC campus made his continued employment at NYCC questionable. His quandary was, in my opinion, an opportunity for the chiropractic program at the University of Bridgeport. Dr. Onorato became the Associate Dean at the University of Bridgeport–College of Chiropractic in June 1992.)

5/16–The letter from the Department of Higher Education was received today.

There is a good possibility we will only be able to accept students who have a baccalaureate degree. Also, we started receiving calls from students wanting information on specific prerequisites explained to them.

I spoke with Ed Eigel who said the state is going out of its way to break balls with their response.

The first checks of the fundraising have started to come in. $750 has been recorded and an additional $500 has been pledged. $1250 so far—it's a start.

(*The response from the state of Connecticut consisted of seven issues which required additional explanation.*)[10]

Issue #1 was an explanation of how the university would control the day-to-day operations of the program; the ownership & control of the university and the governing board. The response consisted of an explanation of how the program, to date, had been developed in conjunction with the university administration and the approval of the University Board of Trustees.

The response also listed the page numbers wherein the names of the University Board of Trustees and administration are listed. Additionally, information was provided in the application about the Chiropractic College Advisory Board. Included in this information were the names of the board members and the bylaws which had been developed by the university attorney and agreed upon by the Advisory Council membership and the university administration.

Issue #2 — addressed contractual relationships of the College of Chiropractic. The response was essentially a repeat of how the college administration would work with the university administration.

Issue #3–The University of Bridgeport must indicate that the program will be supported through its general operating budget–would be the major obstacle in achieving licensure. The response to this issue, though accurate was feeble in light of the money which had been raised by the Genesis Fund Committee. The inability of the university to contribute to or underwrite the proposed college was also problematic.

Issue #4 —addressed faculty credentials and was addressed in the response.

Issue #5 — Admission to a graduate degree program shall require, at a minimum, graduation from an appropriate bachelor's degree program, or the equivalent. Although a lengthy, detailed response was submitted, outlining the admission requirements found in the educational Standards of the Council on Chiropractic Education, this issue would not be addressed until I met with Commissioner Glasgow and her staff at a later date. When the meeting occurred, the information submitted in the application was thoroughly reviewed and found to be accurate. A compromise was agreed upon between the Department of Higher Education and the UB College of Chiropractic to require three years of undergraduate training for students wishing to enter the chiropractic program. The compromise was reached to offset the fact that prospective chiropractic students were not required to take a standardized test like the MCAT.

Issue #6–the involvement of the faculty in the planning of the chiropractic program. My explanation was phrased in a manner which could be understood by educators who had little knowledge or experience with chiropractic education, and as a result it was sufficient to allay this issue. The same could be said for issue #7, which focused on graduation requirements. The response offered was enough to allay the concern of the Department of Higher Education.

Of the seven issues identified by the state, five were addressed by the university response, one (admission requirements) would be addressed in a meeting with the DOE staff, and one (finances) would remain until the end of the licensure process).

5/18–Spent the day working on the response to the state. In addition, I met with a couple of prospective students, one prospective faculty and Walter Wardwell, a sociologist very interested in chiropractic. He has completed manuscript on chiropractic history and is hoping to get it published. In addition he offered his services for the Advisory Board. I will send his résumé and additional information I am accumulating to the Steering Committee.

5/21–Finished the response to the state and gave it to Lillian Nash for typing. If she can have it completed by Wednesday I will get it to Dr. Eigel for re-submission to the state by the end of the week. I would like to have it back by June 1. Aside from that, it was a relatively calm day.

5/23–Between yesterday's phone calls and today's we have surpassed the mark of 200 student inquiries. Spent a great deal of time on the phone with prospective students. The only mail I received was a nasty note from a Connecticut D.C. who indicated he would not be supporting the college because of the D.C.'s on the brochure from NJ and PA. Some people will look for any excuse not to get involved in a positive experience.

5/25–First day of the Memorial Day weekend. Received a call from Stephen Perle, D.C., who wanted to know why there is bad blood between our program and NYCC. He said when Ken Padgett found out about the fundraising brochure, John Danchek was eliminated from the NYCC postgraduate faculty. It is unfortunate that NYCC has such a small parochial view of chiropractic education as to be threatened by our program here at UB.

(Stephen Perle, D.C., would become the first full-time chiropractic faculty member at the University of Bridgeport. At the time of this phone call, he was in private practice and writing a column on Sports Chiropractic for Dynamic Chiropractic. One of his articles titled "University Chiropractic Could Have a Positive Impact" talked of the potential benefits the chiropractic program at the University of Bridgeport might have for the profession.)

Fundraising total as of today, $6500 pledged and $1975 received. The number of student inquiries is 211. In another week after we receive more money I will have applications printed.

Lillian has still not finished the response to the state Department of Higher Education. When completed it will go to Eigel, then John Walters. We need to get this ball rolling and soon.

5/30–Memorial Day weekend was a much appreciated rest. Four more student inquiries today. Received a call from Bob Matrisciano last night. It seems he and several other contributors received letters asking them to donate to the university. Called Bud and informed him of the situation. Marc Peyser will contact Janet Greenwood and find out what is happening. A letter like that could create panic in our prospective contributors.

(The Genesis Fund Committee was having difficulty raising money from the chiropractic profession. The University of Bridgeport was experiencing financial difficulties. The two situations simultaneously were creating a significant obstacle to the completion of this project.)

Lillian Nash gave me the completed version of the state response. I sent it to Ed Eigel and the Steering Committee for their review and comments.

(*The May program updates showed an increase in student inquiries to 209. On the basis of the fundraising brochure being mailed out, $6500 was pledged, with $1975 being received. The State of Connecticut Department of Higher Education responded to our licensure application. A rebuttal was formulated and submitted to the Advisory Council for review and comment. At this point in time, the financial situation for the chiropractic program had become critical. While pledges of money looked good on paper, money was required to complete the assignments necessary for the program to start).* [11]

As of 6/1/90: Applicants
Male–106   Female — 110

State	Number of Applicants	Percentage of Total Applicants
Connecticut	79	37
New York	53	25
New Jersey	32	15
Massachusetts	26	12
Others	26	12

I spoke with John Walters from the state today. He indicated we need to discuss the program. I asked him how many copies of the response he needed. He indicated ten.

Financial calculations as of 6/1/90:
Total Received (by my office) — $37,800
Expenses (Actual)–$36,077.36
Expenses (Estimated)–$1,005.75
Total Expenses — $37, 083.11
Balance — $716.89
The breakdown of expenses is as follows:
Salary — $26,500
Mailing–$9,187.02
Lillian Nash — $139.50
Paper Goods — $159.50

Answering Machine — $91.69_
$36,077.36 (Actual)
Stationery — $350.00
Mail — $115.75
Telephone — $540.00
$1,005.75 (Estimated)

Obviously the program is in dire need of money to keep going. This week we received $275.00. We also have $4900 in pledges. I certainly hope that whoever is supposed to be calling for donations gets going real soon because the money we receive by June 30, 1990, will be the amount by which we are judged by the Board of Trustees. Unfortunately we have gone from a very busy May to a DEAD first week of June. This is not unlike previous slumps, but it would be much easier if we had a financial cushion to live off, at least for the time being.

6/4–I received a call from a Connecticut chiropractor. She had been contacted by Marc Peyser to solicit funds. She received a check-off list of questions to ask but no list of people to call. She informed me that she is going to Ecuador on Friday and will need the balance of this week to focus on personal issues. Therefore she is unwilling to call anyone until she returns on 6/17/90. However, when she returns she will need a week to focus on business. Therefore the earliest she can phone potential contributors is after June 25. If this is the way the fundraising effort is going to be conducted, we have a critical problem.

The brochures have been out for a month and the phone campaign is just beginning. The planning on this phase of the project is to say the least poor. Bob has backed off from his previous efforts because he realized he was the only Steering Committee member soliciting funds.

Received several pieces of mail from prospective students and faculty, but nothing from prospective donors. Some of the mail that came in was postmarked 5/25/90 and I just received it. It takes the mail a week to go from point A to point B in this place. Aside from that it has been a slow day. No prospective students have called for the second consecutive day. It is almost like everyone is watching and waiting to see what happens to the program. I hope we are not entering a death watch.

(The chiropractor contacted to call donors was similar to the chiropractor whose picture was on the fundraising brochure. She was willing to help, but had no idea who to call or what to do. In addition, the Genesis Committee had a hard deadline of June 30 to raise significant money. This individual would be away for most of June, and not be available to start soliciting funds until the end of June. The people trying to raise funds had no idea of the difficulty in getting people to contribute money. They also appeared to have difficulty in communicating. As a result, the program was in grave danger of failing.)

6/6–Busy day. Met with Lyle Hall of Biomedical Models. He showed me anatomical models we might be using in the anatomy curriculum. I calculated the costs of the complete anatomy program and it is estimated at $60,000.

I met with Robert Ortoff of L.F. O'Connell Associates. Marc Dionne with whom I had previously worked is no longer with the company. As a result, the PR information we had developed has hit a snag. Therefore we will have to develop it again.

A prospective student came in and asked questions about the program.

Received a check for $1,000 and brought it over to Mike Bisciglia's office.

With a little luck this could be the best week yet raising money, even though we are a long way from our goal. I can only hope the money starts coming soon.

6/8–Got out report to Advisory Committee. To date we have received about $39,000 with an additional $6,000 in pledges. In the next week I am hoping some significant money comes in. Spoke with another prospective student in person and several on the phone. The only thing we need to succeed is money. I haven't spoken to the Steering Committee members this week. I will give each of them a call on Monday.

6/11–An NYCC representative called and asked if I wanted to sponsor two students at the NYCC Homecoming Banquet. I said no. He shared that morale is bad across the board at NYCC and attendance at Homecoming is really bad. There is little, if any, support from alumni and faculty and there is a strong rumor that a number of third and fourth trimester classes will transfer at the end of this term. According to the rep the situation there has gone from bad to worse. The faculty are upset with Padgett and his intention to turn the school into an ACA based philosophy school only. He wants to eliminate the straight mentality from campus completely. I'm sure the faculty is equally upset that Henry Shull, a former member of the administration has not yet been re-hired by the college. It has been over a year and he is still hanging around. Dr. Padgett maintains he will not hire Dr. Shull back and I'm sure that weakens his standing with some of the faculty.

6/13–Received the "revised" response to the state from Dr. Eigel today. I picked it up at his office at 2:00 p.m. and delivered the completed version to his secretary at 4:15 p.m. In the meantime, I revised the document in the word processor (one paragraph and four words), punched holes in the covers, ran off copies of the response and exhibits, punched holes in the response and exhibits, typed the tabs for the dividers, assembled ten copies of the response and bound each of them. Needless to say the afternoon was quite busy.

Tomorrow I am supposed to go to L.F. O'Connell and see what they have developed in the way of PR to date.

I haven't received anything in the way of money this week.

6/20–For the past couple of days I have been suffering from the flu. This is the sickest I have been in a long time. Getting back to the university did not make me feel any better. The accounting office does not have a record of any money in our account since 5/31/90. I spent two hours this morning figuring out what the problem is. Now to get the principals together to rectify the problem will take even more time.

I received a call from Carmen Tortora, a UB board member who wanted to know if we were going to receive any kind of money to save this program. He instructed me to call one Elliot Konig. I called Marc Peyser and asked that he call Mr. Konig.

6/22–I feel much better today, almost back to normal. Sent the program update to all concerned parties. The chiropractic college is a political football with the winner being the person who makes it go or brings it down, depending on whose side you are on. Janet Greenwood, university president is for the program. The Chairman of the Board of Trustees, Nicholas A. Panuzio, is against the program. If the program fails, I think Jan Greenwood will be fired. If the program succeeds, I think Mr. Panuzio will be ousted as Board Chair. Politics seems to be a way of life in higher education. Unfortunate but true.

State	Total number of prospective students (To Date) (% of total)
Connecticut	83 (35%)
New York	54 (25%)
New Jersey	38 (16%)
Massachusetts	26 (11%)
Rhode Island	5 (2%)
Pennsylvania	5 (5%)
All others	21 (9%)
TOTAL	237

Donations

State	Number of Donors	Receive (in dollars)	Pledged (in dollars)
New York	42	29,100	1,000
Connecticut	9	8,600	5,500
New Jersey	3	2,650	0
Florida	5	675	1,000
Massachusetts	5	625	1,000
Pennsylvania	1	500	1,000
Rhode Island	1	200	
TOTAL		42,320	9,500

All we need are several big donations and the program will be secure.

6/25–This is going to be THE week. Unless we come up with a significant amount of money, as per our agreement (6/30/90), I don't know what the fate of the program will be.

I really can't understand what the rush is concerning funds for our program. It seems that with the financial crunch the university is currently experiencing, it would be better for all concerned parties to exercise patience. The fact that this is not the case indicates to me there is something more than meets the eye going on here.

Reviewed tally sheet from week ending 6/22/90 which reflects revenue received $46,170. Today we received an additional $1300, plus an endorsement from the New England Chiropractic Council. A Connecticut business man called and stated he would be making a large contribution to the program. In addition, Carmen Tortora pledged $20,000 and stated he would pledge an additional amount at a later date. Between what has been received and pledged the total in the Chiropractic College Fund stands at $88,470. If the board is looking to pull out of this program now, there is more happening than we were led to believe originally. However, given the financial condition of the university, I am hoping they will see the wisdom of going along with us.

6/27–Spent the day corresponding with Mike Bisciglia in terms of pledges, prospective students and Carmen Tortora. Tonight I will speak before the Northern New Jersey Chiropractic Association and hopefully collect some money. Between what we have received and what has been pledged, the fund now stands at over $90,000. What we need is a couple of mega-gifts and we will be home free.

I found out that Bob Green, the bursar, resigned and will be leaving in two weeks. Lillian Nash also told me there is a pool betting on when Dr. Greenwood will be leaving the university. If she leaves our program is in big trouble. I can only hope we can accumulate the kind of money we need to keep our program afloat before anything like this happens.

6/29–Spoke at the Northern New Jersey Chiropractic Association meeting on Wednesday night and received a check for $2500, the initial payment of a $5,000 pledge from the United Chiropractic Provider Network. Right now we have received $51, 020 with an additional $44,450 in pledges totaling $95,467. Now all we need are a couple of large contributions and we'll be home free.

Met with a prospective student who seemed genuinely impressed with my description of the program as well as the curriculum. The month of June was slow for prospective students, but I think that can be attributed to the time of year.

I heard that John Fitzpatrick, NYCC's Director of Admissions, resigned. That should help their program. I also heard the new rumor at NYCC is that Mr. Faust will be named VP of Student Affairs and Mark

Feldman, D.C., will be named Dean of Students. That should help their program. In the meantime, we are still awaiting word from the state on our licensure application.

(The administrative changes at NYCC are right out of Keith Asplin's letter to the Board of Trustees regarding the staff changes that undermined his administration. Dominic Fiorello and Stephen Faust were both PhDs and were named to key positions in Academic and Student Affairs. Both had experience in these areas.)

If the rumors I hear are true and Jan Greenwood leaves the university, and Ed Eigel ascends to the presidency, I wonder how supportive he is of the chiropractic program. If he's not, we could be in big trouble.

(The June program updates indicate an increase in student inquiries to 237. The amount of money received in the Chiropractic College Fund rose to $45,000. By this time 49 individuals had made contributions. None of the major contributors the committee had expected to donate had materialized. There was still no plan on the part of the committee on how to raise the money needed. There was also a minimal amount of communication occurring among the committee members so the project was dependent on whatever money could be secured from donors who believed in the value of affiliation of a chiropractic program with a university. The response to the state report was submitted to the Advisory Committee for their review).[11]

7/2–Beaucoup calls today–all wondering about the status of our licensure. If we do not soon hear from the state, I don't think we will be opening in January.

Word out of New York is that we are broke and John Fitzpatrick is back as director of admissions at NYCC.

Aside from that, all is quiet.

(It seemed personnel at NYCC were watching the progress at the University of Bridgeport as closely as I was monitoring what was happening on their campuses.)

7/6–Slow day–slow week with regard to student inquiries. As a matter of fact, this is the worst week we have had since we started this effort.–one inquiry. I received a call from Arnold advising me to send the article I wrote and the press release from the New England Chiropractic Council to *Dynamic Chiropractic*. I hope he finally prints some of this information. I think the reason we are so slow is because July 4 fell in the middle of the week. Some people had off before the holiday, some after. No matter what, July is a slow time of year in any school.

I haven't spoken to Bob Matrisciano in two weeks. Money from New York has dried up and I don't know what is happening. One thing is certain, if it had not been for the money Bob raised to start the program, we would not have gotten this far. I can only hope the July lull that seems to have affected everyone's interest in the program has affected him and that it will pass. I hope things start turning around next week.

(*A program update, 7/6/90, indicates that New York is responsible for approximately 30% of the money received to date. It is also responsible for approximately 1% in pledges to the program. The report also states that approximately two months after the fundraising brochure had been mailed out, the Genesis Fund had not received a single contribution from Vermont, New Hampshire or Maine. There are Genesis Committee members from New Hampshire and Maine and still no results achieved.*

The Advisory Council members were reminded of additional issues which needed to be addressed including: renovation of the anatomy lab, adding membership to the Advisory Council, nominating a dean. All of which needed to be done before the end of the summer).[12]

7/11–Received a call from Ed Eigel's office that the meeting with the Department of Higher Education regarding our license will be next Wednesday at 10:00 a.m. Several more student inquiries received today. I received a call from Arnold who informed me that at the meeting of the Bloomfield College pre-chiropractic Advisory Committee Mort Steuer announced the formation of a new chiropractic college. Principal players in the school would be in addition to Steuer, Jim McDonnell, Frank Langilotti, Don Gutstein and Frank DeGiacomo. This information was relayed by Frank Zaccaria. The plan was not well received by the Bloomfield board.

(*.The North American College of Chiropractic was an idea hatched by individuals who wanted to maintain a chiropractic educational institution in downstate New York. The originators of the school, all severe critics of Ernest Napolitano, now would have the opportunity to run their own program. This was the first and only mention I ever heard of this venture. It was* *a great idea that could not be sold to whomever was needed to establish the funding. Donald Gutstein had served as the Director of the Greenvale Clinic and eventually became a faculty member at Life College of Chiropractic. Jim McDonnell had been released by Keith Asplin and was no longer involved in chiropractic education. Frank Langilotti had distinguished himself during the Trustees conflict as siding with the Clinic Masters block and served as vice president for a day. He returned to work at NYCC in an adjunct capacity until the college moved to Seneca Falls. Frank DeGiacomo remained affiliated with NYCC as a member of the faculty until the school moved up to Seneca Falls. Morton Steuer also remained affiliated in some administrative capacity with NYCC while it remained on Long Island. The document which announced the formation of the college was promoted as a not-for-profit New York state corporation. The information distributed at the Bloomfield College pre-chiropractic meeting was dated October 5, 1991 even though the pre-chiropractic meeting was conducted in July 1990. The obvious purpose of announcing the intentions of the organization was to garner support, both emotional and financial.*

According to the pamphlets distributed at the meeting, the Friends of the North American College of Technology, Inc. was formed to establish a chiropractic college in the metropolitan New York area. In addition, the members of the corporation have entered into extensive dialogue with officers of the New York Institute of Technology to establish a chiropractic college on the central Islip campus of N.Y.I.T. Members of both organizations, according to the informational pamphlet had already met with members of the Department of Higher Education to initiate the process of securing a charter from New York State. Preliminary discussions to outline the steps required to secure a state charter, while a necessary step in the process, does not guarantee the ultimate achievement of the goal.

The Founding members of the Friends of the North American College of Chiropractic. Inc. included Morton Steuer, James McDonnell, Frank langilotti, and Salvatore Curreri, all Doctors of Chiropractic.

The Steering Committee of thwe organization included, Alice Armstrong, John Bonsignor, Paul Cadolino, D.C., Jack Camarda, D.C., Frank DeGiacomo, D.C., Lawrence DeMann, D.C., Donald Gutstein, D.C., Ronald Modesto, Ph.D., Alan Pressman, D.C. and Nathan Washton, EdD, all for-

mer faculty members or staff at the New York Chiropracticd College. The Steering Committee also had several members who were alumni of NYCC.

A second pamphlet describing the Mission, Purpose, Goals and Objectives of the college was also distributed. The contact person listed on this pamphlet was Dr. Morton D. Steuer.

According to the original pamphlet additional news would be forthcoming in the upcoming months on the progress made by the Friends of the North American College of Chiropractic, Inc. and The North American College of Chiropractic.

Dr. Napolitano had secured an absolute charter from the state of New York in 1979, after being affiliated with the New York Institute of Technology for six years. Nappy understood the mechanisms of New York state politics and knew it would require time to secure the goal of an absolute charter. He also understood the educational goals which needed to be secured in the process.

The founding members of the Friends of the North American College of Chiropractic, all critics of Ernest Napolitano, knew what goals would need to be achieved to provide the new college credibility, but they were unable to achieve basic results in their quest. While there may have been many people who wanted a chiropractic college in the metropolitan New York area, funding never materialized. As a result, none of the subsequent goals were ever achieved.

The October 5, 1991 "announcement" regarding the Friends of the North American College of Chiropractic, Inc. was the only information about the project ever disseminated. Frank Zaccaria was a former faculty member at the Columbia Institute of Chiropractic. He was also the treasurer of the NYCC Alumni Association and one of the initial appointees to the Dean's Advisory Council at the University of Bridgeport–College of Chiropractic.)

Sent out pictures to *Dynamic Chiropractic* on Monday for use in a feature article. Actually, I sent out slides because there were no pictures available.

7/12–Spoke to a group of Brooklyn chiropractors last night. They seemed very supportive of our efforts. Gerry Stephens and Alex Pireno were there and I know they are supportive.

7/13–The meeting with State Ed. was changed to 7/12/90 at 9:00 a.m. Received a call from a chiropractor in Indianapolis, Indiana who indicated a desire to get involved on the Advisory Committee. I will send information out to him. I called Marc Peyser and asked him to check this guy out. He called back to tell me this guy is a loser. He said he would call him anyway. Marc also asked me to arrange a meeting with the three wise men for 7/24/90. We need to discuss who should be added to the committee as well as who to nominate for dean and other projects. I certainly hope I can get this meeting off the ground and address these issues.

7/16–Slow, hot, muggy day. We did pick up three more inquiries. I hope some money came in last week and will continue to come in.

7/20–Picked up a few more student inquiries today, the number now stands at 255. Made an appointment to speak at the Nassau Community College Pre-Chiropractic Club on October 4, 1990. Carmen Tortora called—I was out. I have been unable to reach him back. I'm sure he wants to know how the money is coming. Besides that I re-acquainted myself with the material we will be reviewing with the state when we meet on Monday. I spoke with Dr. Eigel's secretary and everything is a go! I only hope our Monday meeting goes well.

7/23–Met today with Dr. John Walters of the state Department of Higher Education. His questions touched upon the curriculum and faculty, but also and most importantly finances. Plain and simple, if the money is not in place prior to commencing the program, the state will not license the program. I spoke with the principals involved and the impression I get is the program is in big trouble. What we need is a miracle. If the article I submitted to *D.C.* comes out in two weeks perhaps it will motivate people to contribute, but in general, I think this project is dead.

Walters indicated a team will come down to campus and address the areas of curriculum, faculty, facilities and library. He also wanted to know if we had checked with the Department of Health regarding cadavers.

Walters wanted to know who is in control of the budget and what provisions are available should the program experience a shortfall. He indicated we should get vitae on clinical faculty. He asked for the names of chiropractors who could serve on the team. He mentioned Bill Fuller as someone who might possibly be on the team because of his experience with chiropractic education.

7/25–Received a call from President Greenwood requesting an update on funding, with a copy to go to Carmen Tortora. September entering class at NYCC will not be full and things are not well in terms of morale. Put together the list of team members for John Walters and gave him a call. He was not in but will call back.

Was notified about a meeting next Tuesday night at Il Bochetto. Received the finished admission applications—they look good. Received a call from L.F. O'Connell regarding their proposal. Money continues to come in at a slow pace. Next Tuesday night's meeting will tell the tale.

7/27–As of today we have accumulated $101,370 in donations and pledges. Of the total, we have received $55,420. We also have accumulated 263 student inquiries.

An article appeared in *D.C.* magazine yesterday which caused a stir at NYCC. I think they are very sensitive now because there projected enrollment for September is less than originally estimated. All in all, today has been rather upbeat considering I wasn't paid again.

(As a response to President Greenwood's request for an update on fundraising and what appeared to be incessant pressure by the Board of Trustees I drafted a letter to President Greenwood wherein I outlined the challenges facing the chiropractic program because of the finances of the university. Also cited in the letter was the adversarial relationship between the administration and faculty.

I then outlined the appeal of the program to prospective students and the potential for revenue. The progress made with regard to our application. We would host a site team from the state on 8/24/90. The fact that efforts to date had not cost the university any money and how the establishment of the College of Chiropractic would address some questions faced by the university going forward.

As a result of this letter, a meeting was held on 8/14/90 between the UB administration and the Chiropractic College Committee. Present at the meeting were: President Greenwood, Provost Eigel, Vice President Beecher, Dr. Cianciulli, Dr. Peyser and myself.

At this meeting (for the first time) I became aware of the reason for the board's impatience with the chiropractic project. The Chiropractic College Committee was to have contributed $200,000 of the $1 million raised to the *general operating fund of the university by June 30, 1990. The inability of the College of Chiropractic Committee to deliver on its fundraising efforts, for one reason or another, had eroded the board's confidence in the project.*

Dr. Greenwood, who was scheduled to address the Pennsylvania Chiropractic Society that weekend, suggested the committee approach ten chiropractors and make each one of them responsible for soliciting $100,000 for the project.

(This proposal was pure fantasy in my mind. The Genesis Fund Committee had not raised $100,000 collectively, I doubted their ability to identify individuals skilled at fundraising.)

In addition, the upcoming site team evaluation was discussed and Dr. Greenwood advised those present that a "serious" offer had been made to purchase the nursing building. As a result, Dr. Zolli was directed to perform a space utilization analysis and determine if the College of Chiropractic could possibly fit into another building.

Dr. Greenwood re-affirmed her commitment to the chiropractic college and reiterated her desire that it should be operational January 1, 1991.

7/30–Called John Walters and gave him the name of four chiropractors:

Milton Meyer (NY)   Paul Grimieson (CT)
William Cirino, Jr. (NJ)   Neil Stern (TX)

Each of these individuals I knew and trusted. They would serve on the state site team. Dr. Walters indicated he had contacted a VP down at Life Chiropractic College who declined participation on the site team due to a scheduling conflict. Spent the day running copies of the original submission plus exhibits and the rebuttal submission. We needed an additional five copies which are now complete. I also went over to admissions and picked up six graduate admission catalogues.

The evaluation visit is tentatively scheduled for August 24, 1990. Dr. Walters indicated he will call me by Wednesday to confirm the arrangements.

Spent the balance of the day prepping for tomorrow night's meeting. Reviewed every topic from finances through accreditation and correspondence. I don't know what's on tap for tomorrow night, but something has to give—soon!

(The July program updates indicate the number of student inquiries to be 256. The amount of money collected by the Genesis Fund stood at $51,620 with an additional $46,700 in pledges. We would be hosting a site team visit from the state on 8/24/90). [13]

8/1–Meeting last night went pretty much as expected. We don't have the money we need and don't know where we are going to get it. All agreed my work has been excellent, but that doesn't get the job done. There was discussion about affiliating with an existing school, National or Parker. The general consensus was that National would probably want the action, but right now I'm not sure if anyone would want to touch this mess.

Spent the morning composing a letter on our finances to Janet Greenwood. The Board of Trustees is really on her ass about this program. I don't know what other issues she is facing right now, but if this program falls flat, it may mean her ouster.

Another option discussed last night was affiliation with Fairfield University. I suppose that can be explored, but I fail to see how a different affiliation will correct the deficiencies exhibited by this crew to date.

8/3–Spent the day preparing the information for the evaluation team. I also made several calls to prospective students. Summertime is slow, but things have picked up here quite a bit. For instance, this week we passed 270 inquiries. The top four states are:

$$CT- 95$$
$$NY- 64$$
$$NJ- 44$$
$$MA- \underline{33}$$
$$236$$

87% of the total number of inquiries. I am unaware of money which has or has not been received this week. I won't receive an update until next Wednesday. Dr. Walters has not called to confirm the date of the visit. If I don't hear from him today, I will call him on Monday. I also want to know who the members of the team will be.

8/8–Met with Ed Eigel to review information for the evaluation team scheduled for 8/24. I had accumulated all the data, wrote a cover letter and sent five packets to Joan Formanack (Dr. Eigel's secretary). I hope she mails this material out today. I also sent this information to the Advisory Committee. I hope things pick up between now and the visit. I scheduled a meeting with Janet Greenwood for next Tuesday. I need to clarify our position here at the university. Rumor has it the nursing building has been sold for $1.3 million. If this is true, we need to move into a different facility on campus.

8/10–Spent the day working on numbers and compiling information for the evaluation visit in two weeks. The packets were already mailed to the team members. The final details regarding the conference room, food, schedule, etc. will be addressed next week. Had a long talk with Bob Matrisciano today. His enthusiasm for the project has definitely waned as a result of the poor communication and follow-through exhibited by the other committee members. He feels the only way to salvage the program is by "selling" it to an established school. He feels it would be difficult to approach Logan. The only viable choices in his mind are National and Parker, although he would not be opposed to approaching Logan. He indicated Bea Hagen is under the gun at Logan and there is a growing sentiment for change at the highest level at that school.

I spoke with Arnold and he feels "selling" is definitely a viable alternative for this project, the only question is to whom? He feels National is our best choice. The entire project hinges on our ability to "sell" this concept to an established school. If and when we do that, there is a distinct possibility that none of the original players, including myself, will be retained. Once another established school is approached, there is nothing to prevent them from approaching the university directly and making a deal on their own. UB needs the money. They will cut whatever type deal is necessary which will ensure funding for the chiropractic program and indirectly, the general operating fund of the university. I only hope the Advisory Committee addresses this issue more thoroughly and vigorously than they have this entire project to date.

8/13–Relatively quiet day. Several calls to NYCC—all quiet there. Three calls from prospective students, total now 278. Received a call from president's office confirming tomorrow's meeting. Now all I have to do is pray the meeting goes well and this program will continue.

8/14–Meeting with Greenwood went well. Minutes put in file for distribution to Advisory Board.

8/15–I met with the university librarian Judith Hunt who seems very pleasant and cooperative. Sent out the minutes from yesterday's meeting to all concerned. I called John Walters to make arrangements for breakfast and lunch for the evaluation team. He advised me to have both served in the team room. Called special services to make all the arrangements. I ordered coffee/tea, pastries in the morning for 12. For lunch I ordered a cold cut platter, condiments, fresh fruit platter, coffee/tea and soft drinks for seven. I calculated it should cost us about $125. For both, I alerted Catherine Yang the invoices would be coming through the system. I picked up the floor plans for north and south halls. I also picked up travel vouchers for the evaluation team.

8/17–I arrived at the office early and was on the go all day. I started off by answering correspondence, then I went over to look at north and south halls in the event the program needs to be relocated to these facilities. I then met with Alan Longerdyke to discuss dormitories. I went with Alan and inspected Bodine and Warner Halls. I would prefer the college be housed in Bodine Hall. The basement can house a variety of labs. The first two floors can be used for offices and classrooms. The balance of the building will be used for dormitory living. It has its own fenced in parking area. This building was closed in May, so the only renovations needed would be cosmetic. Warner Hall is in need of a LOT more work and is an odd-shaped building. When I got back into the office I called Pat Walsh who is writing a speech for Janet Greenwood to deliver this weekend at the Pennsylvania Chiropractic Convention.

(*At this time, due to the decrease in students, the university was in the process of closing dormitories. Bodine Hall was a potential option for the chiropractic building because it had not been closed too long. It also provided sufficient space to house various elements of the program. Warner Hall had been closed much longer and had not been shuttered correctly, as a result pipes had broken in the walls and there was significant water damage throughout the building. It was eventually renovated years later and became the Health Science Center at the University of Bridgeport*).

8/20–Very busy day. This morning I reviewed the floor plans for Bodine Hall. I will walk through the building again on Wednesday. I spoke a prospective faculty member. He is a PT who is currently attending National. Picked up transcripts for two more students and five more prospective students called pushing the inquiry number up to 287. It would be great if we could have 300 by Friday. I wrote a long letter to the son of the business man who indicated he would make a sizeable donation to the college. Hopefully his father will donate $1,000,000 and secure the future of the program. I tried contacting Deans Nechascek and Blackshaw and Rose Galiger without success. The balance of the day was spent answering correspondence. I responded to a letter from SORSI and concluded my response with a request for a donation. It's getting easier to ask for money, now all we need to do is get it.

8/22–I spoke with Janet Greenwood today about her trip to Pennsylvania. She said she had an interesting trip. She received a $5,000 check from the Pennsylvania Chiropractic Society and informed me that Mark Feldman, D.C., from NYCC made several derogatory comments about me. I advised Jan I would respond to Dr. Feldman by letter. After concluding our call I wrote a good letter to Mark which he should receive early next week. President Greenwood also asked me to draft a letter to President Padgett regarding the situation. Spent the balance of the day responding to student inquiries and making last minute arrangements for the evaluation team visit on Friday. I met with Ed Eigel regarding the visit and he feels we are ready.

8/23–I arrived at the office and typed the letter to Ken Padgett that President Greenwood requested. I called a Connecticut D.C. to ask if he would be available to speak with members of the evaluation team. He agreed. I spoke with Lance Blackshaw about the visit and he agreed to give the team a tour of Dana Hall. I spoke with Joe Nechasek and he agreed to meet with the evaluation team about the program. I reviewed the faculty files and selected a representative group to show the team. I typed up the list of faculty and their credentials to have ready for the visit. I went to the library to make sure the conference room was ready. I found out that Judith Hunt had been out sick but will be available tomorrow. I called special events to confirm the food arrangements for tomorrow. I walked over to the nursing building to make sure the rooms were prepared for tomorrow. I mapped out future plans on the floor plans of both

Bodine Hall and the nursing building. I made arrangements to have the keys for both buildings. I made arrangements with security regarding the alarms in the nursing building. Called Mike Bisciglia's office to tell him the name of the president of the Pennsylvania Chiropractic Society.

8/24–The day we entertained the evaluation team from the State of Connecticut Department of Higher Education was a gray, rainy day. Breakfast and lunch went great, right on schedule. For the most part, the team stayed in the conference room and grilled Ed Eigel and me. They then moved on to Dean Nechasek, Dr. Levine and me. The person who most antagonistic and hurtful to us was Gary Johnson, D.C., from Logan College. He was obviously upset about the Advisory Board and the lack of a job description for the position of dean. His overall demeanor was negative. Dr. Walters from the state Department of Higher Ed appears to be interpreting the letter of the law as it pertains to our program. He also indicated it is doubtful we will be on the agenda for the October meeting of the Board of Governors (BOG). I will need to speak to Ed Eigel about applying some pressure to the BOG. The other team members were George Clark and Bill Fuller. George Clark was very reasonable and Bill Fuller was great. After we toured the facilities Bill asked me to drive him to his car. He confirmed my suspicions about Gary Johnson, going so far as to tell me he wants to be the dean of this program. Gretchen Hammerstein, the librarian on the team seems to be a typical librarian. The exit report primarily focused on the clarification of the supervision of faculty, faculty contribution toward curriculum development and the F-word, finances. Bill Fuller indicated the emphasis on finances was not so much related to our program but the overall stability of the university. Now I need to rest.

Next week I will compose thank-you letters to all the appropriate people who made the evaluation team visit a success. I will compose a report to the Advisory Board telling them what transpired today and start working on areas the team felt needed improvement. According to Dr. Walters, the proposal is appropriate and the curriculum is a basic format for a chiropractic curriculum.

8/27–Fairly productive day. Wrote an article which will, hopefully, appear in *D.C.* magazine. Picked up two more potential students. Started working on descriptions for the new members of the Chiropractic College Advisory Board.

(August correspondence indicates the Genesis Fund, in terms of money received and pledges exceeded $100,000. Unfortunately, the Chiropractic College Committee had committed to contribute $200,000 to the general operating fund of the University by June 30. Members of the Advisory Committee were invited to the site team visit on 8/24. None were available to attend. The visit occurred on a Friday, when each of the members practiced. To me, this was further evidence the members of the committee had lost their enthusiasm and commitment to the program. Each of the members knew about this visit and its importance for several weeks, yet they made no effort to alter their schedules.)[14]

9/5–Faculty and several other unions went on strike. The question is, which side can hold out longer? Obviously both sides will be hurt in the process, but a prolonged strike could adversely affect the financial recovery plan of the university. Caught up on correspondence. Students are starting to call and ask about when we will be opening. I sent a financial report to the Advisory Board. If we don't come up with some money soon, we won't have to worry about the university, its politics or anything else. We won't have a school. Passed the three hundred mark in student inquiries on Friday. The number is currently 304.

9/7–The university is still on strike. That means services are less efficient than they usually are. In short, services have gone from bad to worse. I think one of the drawbacks to growth is that things become less personalized and people start to not care. I think the university is filled with this kind of blasé and apathy. I finished the letter Mark Peyser asked me to write to corporate sponsors. I hope this helps the fundraising process. If we don't get a substantial amount of money soon we are going to be out of business.

(The effort for corporate sponsorship was a harebrained scheme devised by the Advisory Committee. I was to write a letter about the program. The letter was to be sent to "select" corporations, and large donations would be forthcoming. This idea was as effective as every other idea which had been formulated by the committee.)

9/17–I haven't made an entry in this diary in over a week because there has been nothing to record. The status of the strike is the same—it is on with no end in sight. For the first couple of days there was no picketing, but since Monday there have been picketers all over, blocking driveways and access to buildings. Lillian Nash's son was arrested for trying to cross a picket line. Actually, he was arrested for mouthing off to a policeman, but Lillian was very upset. Later in the week his car was fire-bombed and Lillian has been receiving lots of nasty phone calls. Lillian told me Catherine Yang resigned today. There has been quite a drop in the number of personnel in the past year. Rumor has it the university is contemplating seeking Chapter 11 relief. Here at the Chiropractic College nothing is going on out of the ordinary, except answering calls now centers around how the strike will affect our opening. The fact is, there is no way we can open in January. I sent notification of this nature to the Advisory Board. We do not have the money to order supplies and equipment. At this point in time we have nothing that someone with financing could not buy from the university for a song. We had our chance and failed, miserably. Fundraising has all but stopped, as have telephone calls. I keep trying to assess why we are in this predicament and keep coming back to the attitude of the Advisory Board. They seem to believe the world cannot live without their input, yet they have contributed little in the way of expertise (or money) to this project. On paper we have raised about $200,000, but in reality we have received about $64,000, most of which is spent. Haven't heard from Padgett or Feldman on the letters they received. They will probably not respond at all. We had a little article appear in *D.C.* magazine last week. I hope we get a big article in the next edition. They did ask for my picture, so I'm hoping it comes out this week.

9/19–Spoke with Ed Eigel today and he informed me that there is little if any chance we will be on the BOG agenda until November. That pretty much eliminates a January starting date. I wrote a letter to prospective students. I hope the Advisory Board sees the wisdom of treating our students like people and not chattel. Other than that, the strike lingers on and replacements are being hired. According to Mike Beecher, there are more faculty in the classroom than there are on the picket lines.

9/24–I didn't make an entry on 9/21 because I really wasn't around too much. My cousin Tony Ricciardone died suddenly on Tuesday and from Thursday through Saturday I was focused on helping my cousin Michael, his brother, and Mary, Tony's wife and his children through their ordeal. Without a doubt, it was one of the saddest experiences I have ever endured.

I spoke with Arnold this morning and he informed me they are going to press Konig for some additional funds as soon as possible. (As far as I know, he has pledged money—given nothing!) I'm not sure about the wisdom of pressing for additional pledge money from someone who has contributed nothing.

Aside from that I spoke with prospective students, answered correspondence and caught up on paperwork. We'll see what happens next.

9/26–Met with prospective student (who did enter and graduate from the program). Talked with several other prospective students about the program. As of today we have 320 prospective student inquiries.

At the request of the president, I attended a meeting where she addressed the faculty. Dr. Greeenwood announced that as a result of the situation which has been ongoing since the beginning of September, the budget for the current fiscal year will be balanced. Ed Eigel reported there are 138 faculty working at the university, as opposed to 170 working last year at the same time. Those individuals who have stayed on the picket lines are now without a job. If they want to come back they will be put on a preferential list, but for the time being they are unemployed. Aside from that the balance of the day was consumed with responding to questions by prospective students and faculty.

9/27–Thursday. Came into work to prepare for a three o'clock meeting with the president. I anticipate a good deal of discussion on the finances of the project. I guess I will have to dance quite a bit given the fact that we are about $800,000 short of our projected goal. On a positive note, we have saved $300,000 since I started here simply by not spending at all. It helps to maintain a budget when you have nothing to spend.

(September correspondence showed student inquiries to be at 314. The Genesis Fund had increased to $206,308. Unfortunately, only $65,000 has been received and the balance is in pledges. Due to the lack of funds and the late date of our appearing before the Board of Governors of the Department of Higher Education, I advised the Advisory Committee the opening of the

program should be postponed until April 1991. There is a letter from President Greenwood to Governor O'Neill requesting the licensure of the chiropractic program be expedited to help the fiscal stability of the institution. Also included was a list of pledges which needed to be followed up. The list was sent to Dr. Peyser.)[15]

10/1–I have not been at UB one year and the end seems in sight. The money problem which has plagued us from day one continues dogging us now. I sent a letter to the Advisory Board outlining our current dilemma. In short, President Greenwood wants me to continue planning for January and we don't have the money for any of it. Janet got a call today from BP who informed her that he feels we would not be able to raise the money. She called me and asked that I arrange a meeting with the committee as soon as possible, i.e. tomorrow morning. She also intimated that perhaps she had not made it clear that the licensure of the program needed to be on the agenda of the BOG in October. When she spoke with BP he had told her the licensure question would be on the November BOG agenda. As a result, she assumed I had not conveyed the proper directives to Ed Eigel.

I called Arnold who immediately stated he would be unable to attend tomorrow morning. He is busy and needs advance notice before he can commit to any meetings. He then asked what the meeting was about. When I told him finances. His response, "Did I call Bob?" It's funny, he never calls the people he says he is going to call for weeks at a time. At any rate, the situation is bleak and there is little that can be done without a concerted effort by all involved.

It is impossible to open in January. There is simply too much work undone and no money to do it. A university-based chiropractic program is an idea without much popular support. A good idea plagued by poor financial planning, based on an unstable financial environment, without popular support is a bad idea.

10/3–I received approval from Ed Eigel on the letter I want to send to prospective students. I guess this closes the book on this enterprise, certainly for January. The reality, plain and simple is there was no concentrated effort at getting money. It is apparent Arnold and Bud were banking on Bob Matrisciano to do the job and although he has tried (the only person to do so), the lack of effort by the others, the strike, the bad publicity surrounding UB has all proved to be too much. I finally arranged a meeting with the Advisory Committee and President Greenwood on 10/11/90 at 9:00 a.m.

I wonder if this enterprise will reach a one year anniversary (10/25/90). I have the letters to students ready to be mailed. I will write a separate letter to faculty. Then I will write a press release for *Dynamic Chiropractic*.

It feels good to have something to do every day, but it also feels frustrating to think I am all alone and out on a limb.

10/17–There has been no entry in two weeks. On October 6, 1990, my father passed away. His death was sudden and unexpected. He had been feeling well since his hospital stay in July and in fact complained very little about the arthritis which had plagued him for years in the weeks before his death. After going shopping with my mother, he collapsed at home. My sister Angela attempted to administer CPR while my mother massaged his neck. According to my sister, during this procedure, he opened his eyes, looked at my mother and sister, then closed his eyes and he was gone.

I was home working on our response to the state when I received the call. I rushed to Jersey City with Adelia, but he had already died by the time we arrived. I was impressed by the expression of peace on his face when I first viewed his body. He looked like he was sleeping. When I kissed him, he was still warm, and in my heart I knew, that despite the shock and pain we were experiencing, he was in a better place.

My father always feared doctors and hospitals. He was afraid of dying of cancer, a fate which had befallen his father and two of his brothers. All three of these deaths were long, painful, horrible experiences, so God is just. I am unsure of why my father was taken at this time, but His ways are not meant to be understood. I trust there is a purpose to everything I have experienced since October 6, 1990, and I live each and every day with a new appreciation of mortality and effort.

There is little to say regarding the program. The meeting held on 10/11 between the university administration and the Chiropractic College Committee appears to have yielded progress regarding fund raising. Marc Peyser addressed the CCA in my absence. I have been catching up on correspondence and working on our rebuttal to the state report. I hope to have the response completed by the end of the week.

10/22–26—All this week has been dedicated to formulating a response to the state of Connecticut's site team visit. The final draft will be completed on Monday when I meet with Drs. Greenwood and Eigel. The points the state are really focused upon are: admission requirements, graduation requirements and all aspects of finance. The only critical issue is finances, which continues to plague the entire country at this time.

On Thursday, the first year anniversary of my starting at UB, I visited NYCC to thank everyone for the sympathy and support they expressed when my father passed away. On Wednesday I had called NYCC and spoke with Ken Padgett and asked his permission to visit the school. He willingly approved. As a matter of fact, when I visited campus we shared about 20 minutes together discussing various professional topics. Chiropractic education was not a topic discussed. A lot of new faces at NYCC and the old faces look tired and worn.

On Wednesday I completed the state response and dropped off copies at the offices of Drs. Greenwood and Eigel. Today I met with four students from Life and a prospective student whose husband currently attends Palmer. All the students were genuinely pleased with the progress we have made and are looking for the school opening, whenever.

10/29–The week started with a 7:30 a.m. meeting with the president and provost.

They were minimally critical about the response I had put together to the site team evaluation report. The few areas of concern they voiced were revised throughout the morning and a final version was delivered at 1:00 p.m. for Dr. Eigel's review and approval. On Wednesday I will assemble the reports and deliver them to the provost's office for mailing. Aside from what appears to be my endless involvement with licensure and several calls from prospective faculty, the balance of the day passed in an uneventful manner. One surprise was Adelia calling this morning to wish me luck and tell me she loves me. I am lucky.

10/31–Received Ed Eigel's revisions, made the necessary revisions and copied the necessary documents. The state report is finished. Nine copies were forwarded to the provost's office for distribution to the president, provost, Advisory Council members and the state. I kept one copy for my records. When I called John Walters this morning he seemed confused as to the number he needed. He hesitantly asked for six and I gleefully offered eight.

I am glad work on this report is finished. Now I can start working on other issues such as admissions, financial aid, curriculum and faculty. I will meet with Joe Nechasek on Friday, admissions on 11/19, in addition to meeting with Norma Abrams of Financial Aid and Bob Singletary of Biology. I spoke with Marc Peyser late this afternoon and he advised me he told Keith Overland the project is in financial trouble. I chastised Marc for this foolishness because word will spread around of this nature and second, even if people have money pledged to the program they will be reluctant to donate it to the Genesis Fund if they feel it is going to be lost on nothing. It is frustrating to think I have spent all this time and energy on a program which, contrary to what I was told in the beginning, was a long shot to get started. Now I find the individuals on the committee are the very people working against our getting off the ground. The phone had been quiet this week—now I know why. I also spoke to Bob and Arnold about the situation and Marc's comments. For all intents and purposes they too have given up. Money is the problem and no one on the Advisory Committee knows where we are going to get it.

(Program updates for October advised the committee that Dr. Greenwood directed me to continue planning all phases of the college. Student inquiries now stand at 362. The College of Chiropractic was named the beneficiary of a $25,000 life insurance policy. This was given instead of a large donation which had been expected by the members of the Advisory Council. The final response to the Department of Higher Education in support of our licensure application was sent to the Advisory Council for their review.)[16]

11/2–Met with Joe Nechasek who advised me to contact university faculty to determine if they are interested in teaching in the chiropractic program. He told me to check with Lance Blackshaw for names of chemistry faculty and also announced the air conditioning/ventilation system in the nursing building needs to be repaired.

(A small article appeared in Dynamic Chiropractic under the title, "Chiropractic Gaining Respect at the University of Bridgeport." The article reported

on the August site team visit from the state as part of the licensure process.)

11/15–I haven't made an entry on almost two weeks because it has been quiet for the most part. Last week I was occupied with the death of my Aunt Michaelina, the fourth death in the family since September 18.It's amazing, but as I make this entry it seems the last two months have been a blur. The family lost Uncle Tony (Alexander) Cousin Tony (Ricciardone) my father and now Aunt Mikey (Zolli). Pop would have been proud that at his sister-in-law's funeral three of his children were in attendance. Only Alex, who lives in Ohio was missing.

I spend a lot of time shuttling back and forth to New Jersey trying to bring closure to things my father started, like finding out why Tony Ricciardone's family was not notified about his death by the hospital to which he was taken, and my sister Angela's malpractice suit. This past Tuesday Angela signed a contract with a lawyer and the suit is now on the record. Hopefully in a couple of years it will be settled in Angela's favor.

Yesterday, 11/14/ 90, I received a copy of the state response to my rebuttal of their site team report. The state backed off on ALL issues except one: Money.

(There is a single program update for November which updates the committee on the meetings of the university with the committee on Accreditation of the Board of Governors. The remaining issue, which needs to be addressed by the committee is securing funding.)[17]

11/15–I met with Janet Greenwood, Ed Eigel, Mike Bisciglia and Sara Melendez to discuss the upcoming meeting of the Committee on Accreditation of the Board of Governors. President Greenwood wants overt pressure applied to have the program licensed.[18] Ed Eigel thinks the best thing to do is pull the licensure application from the agenda before it is rejected. Sara Melendez believes it will be rejected solely because of lack of funding. She feels the university should scrap the program and Mike Bisciglia is annoyed the university was led down the primrose path by unsubstantiated claims of financial backing. As he pointed out, the representatives of the chiropractic profession with whom he originally met indicated it would be no problem raising the $1 million dollars required. He also said that several members of the Board of Trustees who contribute to the university's yearly fund resigned from the board because of the university's decision to establish a College of Chiropractic. Now we are saying we cannot raise the money.

Realistically we are $500,000 short of the money needed to get licensed. One of the reasons we need so much money is because the university cannot commit any funds to the project, nor can they underwrite the program in case of a financial shortfall. Their bank will not allow them to incur any debt and it would be political suicide for them to divert funds to support a new school when they have dropped established programs due to financial constraints.

I have thought about this situation often over the last few months and I am amazed we have gotten as far as we have. There are two major problems which have undermined this project from the start. Dishonesty is the first culprit. From day one there has been dishonesty among the primary players.

No one on the chiropractic committee, ever indicated the university was in as bad financial shape as it is. Perhaps they didn't know, but neither did they thoroughly investigate the matter. To make matters worse, the committee negotiated a deal where our school will a) get a second rate building for use and b) split our profits 50/50 with the university. The law school only pays 15%. Finally I think the committee overestimated the support the concept of a chiropractic school becoming affiliated with a university would receive from the chiropractic profession at large. Dr. Matrisciano was able to raise about $30,000 quickly, but put the brakes on when he realized he was the only person raising money. The other members thought that mailing a flyer with their picture on it would be enough to get money into the program. Bob has taken the position that he is not going to risk his neck (and reputation) soliciting funds when nobody else is. Marc Peyser is telling people we need the money and don't have it. When I told Marc this was not a bright comment to make in that people who have pledged money to the program might not donate it now, he said he hadn't thought about that.

So now we face our last hurrah. If we do not receive an infusion of money in the next three weeks the program will not be licensed and the program will be dead. I do not know what this will mean for the university, but for the profession of chiropractic it will be an embarrassment. It will be a personal disappointment and embarrassment for me, but I think it will be worse for the members of the committee who are visible leaders in the profession. I only hope that our failure, if it happens, will not jeopardize future efforts to have a chiropractic program affiliated with a university. It's a great idea whose time has come. Now all that is needed is the right opportunity.

11/16–Today I met with Carmen Tortora for the first time. He was quite displeased that so little had been accomplished by the chiropractors with regard to fundraising. I told him about a charitable trust idea that I hoped would induce him to take advantage of it for himself or sell the idea to some of his wealthy friends. I spoke with him for about an hour. He showed me a fundraising proposal developed by his son-in-law. It is a good proposal but a year too late, which is what I told him.

Mr. Tortora said he wanted to call all the chiropractors in the state and all the vendors who do business with them. I came back to the office, copied the list of D.C.'s, called the CCA for a list of vendors. I was told I would have the list next week.

I received a call from Sara Melendez. We are on the Board of Governors' agenda on Tuesday! It seems the intense lobbying by herself, Jan Greenwood, and Mike Bisciglia has paid off. I don't know what the result is going to be, but if their behind the scenes lobbying is successful, and Janet can reach Norma Glasgow, the Commissioner of Education, perhaps we can pull a rabbit out of the hat. After that, it is anybody's guess as to what will happen. If Carmen Tortora can come up with money, we will be on our way.

11/20–Went to Manchester, CT today for a meeting with the Academic Affairs Committee of the Board of Governors. Sara Melendez accompanied me. We got there in time for the meeting, only to have to wait three hours as the board debated the issue of whether or not Housatonic C.C. should receive a license for the nursing degree program. When we made our presentation, the board listened patiently to John Walters from the state and Sara Melendez from the university. They then asked some questions before deferring their decision for 30 days. On a positive note, John Walters reiterated that there is only one problem with the program, money. We discussed the library and I gave him additional vitae of some prospective basic science faculty. Norma Glasgow, the commissioner of Higher Education, said she was optimistic we would receive licensure after the 30-day deferment period.

11/21–I met with Jim Schenks, Carmen Tortora's son-in-law regarding a marketing plan for fundraising. We met for a couple of hours and hopefully we will have a well thought plan by the middle of next week. Mr. Tortora indicated he knew a business man who would give $100,000 to the program. He indicated an additional $100,000 would be donated by some other foundation he knows. Mr. Tortora himself indicated he would donate an additional $125,000 if we could get half of this pledged money up front. If that occurred we would be in excellent shape!

I still have not received the list of vendors from the CCA. Spoke with Bill Tkacs who told me he would be hearing on Monday about our funding request from Fuji.

(*The Fuji proposal was part of the corporate fundraising scheme thought up by the Advisory Committee. I don't know if it was real. I spoke with Bill Tkacs by phone about the initiative. I was never asked to provide any information about the program to him. My knowledge of the proposal was an occasional call regarding its progress.*

The Fuji proposal, as well as the large pledges from Mr. Tortora's business friend, foundation, and himself never materialized.)

11/22–Thanksgiving Day—the first without my father. The day passed without difficulty. Everyone was hurting, but everyone was hurting together.

11/23–Today I worked on information I will share with Jan Greenwood on Monday. Also I noticed I neglected to make an entry on 11/19. On that day I met with admissions, financial aid, Judith Hunt, the librarian and got everything prepared (faculty vitae for John Walters) for the meeting with the Board of Governors on 11/20. On 11/20 I was up at 5:00 a.m., out of the house by 6:00, picked up Sara at 8:00, got back from Manchester at 4:00, left the university at 5:00 and returned home at approximately 7:00 p.m. Definitely a fun day.

11/28–Since meeting last week with the Board of Governors I have worked on little else except the budget. I have trimmed the proposed budget as much as possible. Because we have no money behind us, we are short by $150,000 I called John Walters who told me what I need to have in the report to the state. I spoke with Sid Kaufman about prices for tables and equipment. Now all we need is the money. Today has not been a particularly good day. I was informed I will not be paid on Friday because there is no money. I have not heard from the committee in some time. They have distanced themselves from this project totally. I'm sure they will be there for the bows, but for now, they are ghosts and I am all alone.

11/30–November ended on a mixed note. I spent the day accumulating information we need for the meeting in Hartford on Tuesday with the Department of Higher Education. One of the pieces of information I received was the account sheet for the program. To date we have spent $66,249.33. The amount of money received in donations is $67,580 which means we have an excess of approximately $1300.00. We received $1800.00 yesterday, which means I might be able to be paid next Friday for work completed in October. I won't complain as long as I continue to be paid.

Received a call to say we have not heard from Fuji. I spoke with Jim Schanks who indicated he will not have the finished proposal until next week. He was basing his timeline on a discussion he had with Carmen Tortora who told him we did not need the information until the middle of December. I spoke with John Walters who wants us to verify pledges. I called Mike Bisciglia to request a written statement and print out of pledges. He indicated that Carmen Tortora had withdrawn his pledge. He also said he had nothing from Eliot Konig to verify a pledge. This is contrary to what I had been told by Mr. Tortora. I called Bob Matrisciano to tell him I had a painting of Dr. Napolitano he could give to Mollie Donovan if she gave the program a big donation.[19]

12/3–Spent the day preparing for our meeting with the Department of Higher Education tomorrow. I have files on library, faculty, including a tentative April schedule of teaching assignments; a phase-in program for equipment, budgets, pledges, fundraising and a copy of the expenses the program has incurred. I need to meet with President Greenwood at her home at 8:00 a.m. for our trip to Hartford. I spoke with Rose Galiger and Mike Autori about teaching in the program. They both seem willing and enthusiastic. I will be meeting tomorrow night at Il Bochetto to brief the committee on the current situation. I still have not heard from Carmen Tortora. By my calculations we are about $50,000 short of opening.

12/4–Met with Norma Glasgow, Mark Johnson, and John Walters of the Department of Higher Education today. They seemed very critical of the last two issues and were not the least bit helpful. Today they were real bureaucrats, not giving definite answers and hiding behind nebulous regulations. The issue of requiring a baccalaureate degree came up again. John Walters is really pushing for it to be a requirement. Hopefully this batch of information, including a thorough narrative, will give us the license we have long pursued.

12/5–Exceptionally busy day. Worked on getting together all the information for John Walters. Completed the work and faxed him the information at 4:00 pm. He had called earlier in the day asking about faculty numbers. I will get that information to him on Friday. I told him we had secured a library consultant, Marilyn Stern, and he was pleased. He advised me how he thought it would be best to present the fund-raising–pledges part of our revenue chart. I called Marilyn Stern and she was thrilled about the opportunity to work as our consultant. As a courtesy, I called Ken Padgett to request that I be able to speak with Marilyn. He was not pleased but he commented that he could not stop anyone from consulting on their own time. He also asked if we would be requiring a bachelor's degree as an admission requirement. I told him the state wanted it as a requirement but we were fighting them on the issue. I spoke with Neil Stern who asked about the program after providing me with costs associated with PG/CE. Aside from that I needed to have copies available for the state, Advisory Board and to Board of Trustees.

12/7–I spoke with John Walters yesterday and he advised me the application would be going to the Academic Affairs Committee again. This means all the material I accumulated has to be mailed out this morning. Upon arrival in the office I typed out the faculty requirements and faxed them to John Walters in Hartford. I called him a little later and asked his recommendations on the material I had submitted today and on Wednesday. He gave me some suggestions. I typed the introduction, table of contents, library section, numbered all the pages then faxed him a completed version. I then wrote a program update for the Advisory

Board and mailed them their monthly packet of information. I spent the balance of the day filing, writing correspondence and reviewing documents of potential students. If and when we receive $150,000 this is going to be a great chiropractic college.

12/10–After hustling all last week to assemble and mail our information to the state, I feel like I'm on vacation with a normal amount of work to do. Yesterday I took Adelia to look at my new office. After it is cleaned up, it should be nice. Now, all I need is some money to make it happen, and it will happen. Things here at the university are bad—cash flow problems are creating major stress. I have heard nothing about our fundraising, which is not a surprise. I'm trying to stay positive about this situation but it is getting more and more difficult, especially with the money crunch being experienced by the university. Arnold called me twice last week and told me how much my efforts have been and are appreciated. I answered and told him I feel like I am out on a limb, all by myself. He assured me I'm not, but the reality is, I am. I got out correspondence and made up requirement checklists for applicants. Tomorrow I am supposed to meet with Richard Coopersmith, the new president of the CCA, to have him look at our facilities for next year's CCA convention. I think I should cancel the meeting until after the holidays.

12/11–Met with CCA reps. They toured the facilities and have decided to hold the spring CCA convention on campus. It is good PR for the program, providing there is a program.

12/12–I reviewed the academic records of prospective students while trying to figure out if I will be getting paid on Friday. I received a call from a New York D.C. who heard the program is dead. So this time I agreed with her, facetiously. If people who know nothing about the program can make pronouncements about its demise and still other people believe them, what can I do? The problem is now, what it was a year ago—lack of money. I have come to the conclusion my colleagues on the Advisory Board never intended to raise money for this venture. They made one feeble attempt at a fundraising drive, but in reality there was never any intention on their part to follow-through. Here is our financing history in retrospect:

1. Originally, a $300,000 trust fund, controlled by a chiropractic supporter, was to be diverted to this program. (The committee thought this was in the bag. They had $300,000.)
2. A Connecticut D.C. had a family whose business would donate $250,000 to the program. What we received was a $25,000 life insurance policy to be paid in the event of the D.C.'s demise. (The committee thought this was in the bag also, now they had $550,000.)
3. A Connecticut D.C. pledged $10,000 in April before the CCA membership. WE never received a penny.
4. Of all the chiropractors whose names and faces went out on the fundraising brochure, none have contributed, except the members of the Advisory Council.
5. Lists of chiropractors with money in the state were to be developed and PERSONALLY contacted by members of the Advisory Board. It never happened.
6. I was told, all we need is 1,000 chiropractors to donate $1,000 each and we would reach $1,000,000. The 1,000 chiropractors were never identified and therefore, never contacted. The money never came in.
7. The original agreement called for the project to be funded by the chiropractic profession. (No one accurately assessed the attitude of the profession regarding this venture.)
8. The committee feels we need an angel, because we will never raise the money from the profession. *(What happened to the previous angel donations? Who is going to identify this angel and more importantly, who is going to be able to get a donation from this individual?)*
9. Marc is telling people, "Without money, we are dead."

   a. Bob has backed off completely realizing these guys don't know what to do or how to do it.
10. Carmen Tortora won't even answer my phone calls.
11. Elliot Konig, another angel, has been a bust.

    b. The university administration has a very low opinion of the committee's analysis of the situation, as does anyone with half a brain.

c. Anyone involved in this project never knew how bad the finances at the university were.

The reality is if we don't get an influx of money (or a miracle), the program is dead. Without money staff cannot be hired nor equipment ordered. Without money we will not be licensed by the state. This was a great opportunity doomed because the people involved didn't understand the environment in which they were playing. They overestimated their own abilities to attract donors and underestimated the obstacles of raising money. That we have progressed this far is a miracle, but the end is definitely in sight.

12/14–Ed Eigel called and told me he had attended the meeting of the Committee on Accreditation of the BOG yesterday. The committee decided to defer licensing the chiropractic program because the university had not committed to underwrite the cost of the program in case of a financial shortfall. He then spoke with Mark Johnson and John Walters who told him if the university agreed to underwrite the program it would be approved. He conveyed that message to President Greenwood who in turn told him to fax a statement to the state confirming the university would support the chiropractic program in case of a shortfall. According to Ed, we should be licensed on Tuesday. He told me to tell the members of the Advisory Council the good news. I called Arnold and he was pleased. He asked me how I felt and I told him licensure means very little because we are broke. He told me I was being unrealistic about the situation and he would check on the Fuji proposal with Marc Peyser and get back to me. This was at 11:45 a.m. I then called Bob and told him the news. He was ecstatic. I also shared with him my sentiments. The problem with the situation is, even if we get licensed, the Executive Committee of the Board of Trustees can pull the plug on the program because we did not keep our end of the bargain. Even when we achieve licensure, we are only halfway there.

Ed Eigel indicated I would need to bring the multiple budgets for the program I had developed to the Trustees meeting on Thursday and explain them.

12/17–Arnold called me on Friday and relayed the Fuji proposal is on the desk of the president of Fuji and he would talk to me about it on Monday. Big deal. Proposals get lost on presidents' desks all the time. We don't have the money, nor do we have a reasonable chance of getting it.

(*I was unaware of why the members of the Advisory Committee put such emphasis on the Fuji proposal. Aside from the fact it would relieve the members of their responsibilities, and it was their last effort at securing funding, I don't know why this "hail Mary" pass was given such importance.*)

I met with two prospective students today, one, who has completed two years of undergraduate study and another who has just completed her first quarter at Life. The first was accompanied by his father, mother and brother. His brother just graduated from NYCC. I advised him to achieve his undergraduate degree, then apply to UB. The second has a B.S. degree and might be able to transfer.

I prepared 159 envelopes and applications to be mailed to prospective students on Wednesday afternoon, provided we still have a program.

12/18–I arrived at Waldemere Hall (UB president's residence) at 8:00 a.m. and met Ed Eigel who informed me that Janet Greenwood's mother passed away and Janet would not be making the trip to Hartford today. We arrived in Hartford after a harrowing trip (rain, slippery) and attended the Academic Affairs Committee meeting. After a little discussion, the program was approved by a vote of 9-0. We then waited until 4:15 for the final vote by the Board of Governors. Dr. Jeremiah Lowney, Jr. (a dentist) asked some exceedingly stupid and picayune questions, all of which had been answered in the licensure application, the site team report, our rebuttal to the site team report and again today before the full board. He was really hammering away at John Walters who glanced over toward me. I felt bad for John and how he was being treated. When Dr. Lowney asked his next unnecessary question I interjected that the information for which he was looking could be found on the specific pages of the various documents that had been submitted. It became apparent to anyone listening to the exchange that Dr. Lowney was either busting balls or had not read the material. At any rate, after this exchange Dr. Lowney backed off. When the vote was taken, the chiropractic degree program of the University of Bridgeport was licensed by the State of Connecticut Department of

Higher Education by a unanimous vote of the Board of Governors.

When I got back to the office I called Adelia to tell her the good news. I called my mother, to share the good news. I called Keith Overland to tell him the wager he has made with me for $1 that we would never be licensed, he lost. (I never collected on the bet, probably because the odds were 1,000,000:1.) I also called Arnold Cianciulli, Bob Matrisciano and *D.C.* magazine.

12/19–I went to the Board of Trustees meeting. Ed Eigel reported on what has transpired regarding the chiropractic program over the last 14 months, including yesterday's events. I then reviewed the budget for the program with them. I was then asked to leave the room. After several minutes Carmen Tortora exited the room and told me the Board of Trustees had voted in favor of opening the University of Bridgeport–College of Chiropractic–the nation's first university-based chiropractic program.

I went back to the office and called Arnold. He was on a long distance call and could not speak with me. I called Bob Matrisciano who laughed and asked me if the board had figured out how they were going to pay for the program. I called Marc Peyser and he asked me what we are doing about the money. Here they are, the Steering Committee of a historic venture, reacting to the accomplishment with the same level of enthusiasm they exhibited while fundraising!

Future Foundation

1/2/91–I have spent the last two weeks renovating my new office in Jersey City. One thing I learned from my NYCC experience is that I need to have an alternate method of making a living outside of education. Between 12/19 and today I mailed out over 160 applications to prospective students. That's $12,000 in application fees if they are all returned. That is a good thing because as of the last Friday in December yours truly is owed $9850 in back pay. In the meantime nothing can be done in terms of creating or ordering catalogues or brochures or equipment or hiring staff. I am tired of being the entire staff. I am tired of being underpaid, or more accurately, not paid. I want to be paid the money I am owed and slip away to private practice. I am tired of being lied to by everyone. At this point in time, I want this nightmare to be over and I want to be left alone.

1/7–Bud Passero had a day I'm sure he would rather forget. He called to wish me Merry Christmas and Happy New Year (I hadn't heard from him in about 6 weeks.) I told him I was not happy and why and he told me he would get back to me. He called back about three hours later and told me to write a letter to the Advisory Council listing the issues that need to be addressed, i.e. expansion of the Advisory Council, selection of the dean, etc. I told him I had sent this information to the Advisory Council last month. He told me Arnold and Marc had not read that report. I went berserk! I told him the Advisory Council members got into this situation as a lark. None of them have taken their responsibility seriously. I reminded him an enterprising school or individual could have this program for $150,000 down from the $1,000,000 originally sought 16 months ago, and now the "owner" would have a licensed program.

Bud said that he didn't think Janet Greenwood would sell us out. I replied she had given the Advisory Board a year to raise the money, and it had failed miserably. As President of the University of Bridgeport, Dr. Greenwood's only responsibility is to act in the best interest of the university. She couldn't care less about who is in charge of the chiropractic program, as long as the program is a source of revenue for the general operating fund.

Furthermore, Bob Matrisciano had been set up by Arnold and him and was not fooled by their plan. In short, they thought he would raise the money (or fund it himself), I would do all the work and they would call the shots. At this point in time, Bob is on the Board of Trustees. As a result he has access to the president and the other members of the board. He wants me to be named dean, and so do I. If this does not happen, he is ready to walk, and so am I.

Once the dean is selected by the president, he/she will have all the power of running the program and the Advisory Board will have little if any. That's why it is important for the right individual to be selected as dean. The wrong person can undo all the work that has gone into creating the program, and indirectly affect chiropractic education and the chiropractic profession in an adverse manner. Our phone conversation was over.

I also spoke with Jim Schanck, Carmen Tortora's son-in-law who is looking to get paid for the proposal he developed. He spoke with Carmen who told him to call me and keep track of whatever time he is putting in—he will be paid. Jim was shocked to find out that I am owed two months back pay and his father-in-law has yet to come through on money he pledged to the program. (I did not tell him his father-in-law had withdrawn his pledge.) Jim told me he would keep in touch, and if we ever get money, he is willing to work with us.

A program update report, dated January 7, 1991, was forwarded to the members of the Advisory Council. In it Dr. Zolli explained the positive action by the Board of Governors, as well as the subsequent action by the UB Board of Trustees voting the following day to establish the nation's first university-based chiropractic degree program. As part of this action, Robert Matrisciano, D.C., was appointed to the Board of Trustees of the University of Bridgeport.

The balance of the report was a list of assignments which needed completion:

The library plan which had been recommended by the State of Connecticut Department of Higher Education

Renovations to the anatomy complex and the development of brochures and public relations material

Ordering equipment and placing book orders

Proceeding with the fundraising proposal which had been submitted to the state.

All projects were placed on hold due to lack of funding.

The report went on to read, "... the actions of the Advisory Council, though well-intentioned, have been erratic and ineffective. Their lack of resolve in addressing the operational planning and fundraising components of the program have, in effect, crippled the program."

Dr. Zolli went on to suggest actions to jump-start the program.

The appointment of Dr. Matrisciano as Chair of the Advisory Council.

Meeting with Dr. Overland, the president of the Connecticut Chiropractic Association, to start the process of selecting a dean for the college.

Define the requirements for new members of the Advisory Council.[1]

1/9–I sent out ten more applications. Made an appointment to meet with Fran Pichard to discuss our feature article in *D.C.* I also spoke to Jeff Lockheart about the Charitable Lead Trust. I will get this information to Bob on Friday. Bud still hasn't called back, I wonder why?

1/14–I met with Lyle Halls and Peter Galton regarding the purchase of anatomical models for the anatomy lab. I met with Bob Singeltary, chairman of the Biology Department to discuss the renovation of Dana Hall and how it will impact our respective programs. I offered a proposal to allow their transitional physiology laboratory, to be housed in our building, used for all physiology courses. I want there to be cooperation between the College of Chiropractic and the other university programs once we get off the ground.

1/16–I met with Helen Burland to discuss the university admissions office and how it might help the chiropractic program. I met with Norma Abrams about financial aid and Francine Pichard regarding public relations for the program.

(After meeting with Helen Burland and watching the operations of the admissions office, I decided the College of Chiropractic had to have its own admissions staff.)

1/18–Received an interesting call from Bob Matrisciano. It seems Arnold called him to inquire about who he would recommend from New York to work as a consultant for Arnold's IME company. At the same time he informed Bob that he had invited George McAndrews and Don Peterson, Jr. to become members of the Advisory Board. Bob is very upset. He has been talking with people about becoming members of the Advisory Board *after* they contribute money to the program and Arnold is giving seats away to people whom he knows. There has apparently been no change in the attitude of some individuals associated with this project, even after all that has transpired. Bob is discouraged, as am I. Bob has known from the beginning of this enterprise that he was being used simply to get money, and the decisions would be made by Arnold, Bud and Marc. Arnold confirmed this suspicion today by adding members to the Advisory Council. When I spoke to Arnold I relayed this information to him. Arnold responded that he was sorry he ever got involved with Bob in this venture. He feels Bob is too negative and many people do not like him. The translation: Bob cannot be handled by Arnold.

The reality is, Bud, Bob and Arnold each have naysayers attached to them. You cannot ascend to a position of political power, which each of them has, without making enemies. Arnold dismisses these criticisms against him and Bud, but not Bob. I then told Arnold I cannot keep coming to the university without being paid. His response, "You can't get blood out of a stone." He further stated that I should not go up there, check my phone messages by remote, and make arrangements to conduct whatever business is necessary by phone. Arnold does not have the slightest idea of the complexities required to plan and maintain a program. Forget about Bud or Marc, they appear to know less than Arnold.

In retrospect, I feel like a fool. I have known Arnold since I was in grammar school He has been my mentor through chiropractic school and practice. He has been my role model and friend. When Dr. Napolitano announced I had betrayed him, it was Arnold who stood by me and told Nappy I was not a traitor. In this instance, he had been less than honest with me numerous times. He used me.

While I came to know Bud through Arnold, he too became somewhat of a friend and role model. This is the first time I ever worked with him so closely. This has been a giant disappointment. Not only did he make outrageous promises about funding to the university, he was less than honest with me. As a matter of fact, both he and Arnold are guilty of the same sin.

Although I'm sure Bud and Arnold discussed this matter between themselves, their assessment of the situation was as follows: Money was going to be easy to secure, so in effect all they would need to do is sit back and call the shots. Bob, who is known to have money and position in New York, was enlisted to donate money and solicit money. New York is the largest state in the tristate area, with the most chiropractors. The reason Bob was nominated for the Board of Trustees is because trustees are expected to be large contributors to the university. That gives you an indication of their ignorance with regard to university politics. As a trustee, Bob will have access to the board and university administration. As members of the Advisory Council, they have access to the Dean of the College of Chiropractic. Bob is in a better position to remove them from the equation then they are to remove him.

Which leads us to the Advisory Council, a committee whose function is misunderstood by Bud and Arnold. The Advisory Council is meant to advise the Dean on professional issues. It is not a substitute for the Board of Trustees. I believe Bud and Arnold think they will position a candidate of their choice in the position of dean, then control the operations of the college from behind the scenes.

They have outsmarted themselves this time. Yesterday, Arnold questioned how Bob could be a trustee at Logan and UB simultaneously. It's simple really. The CCE standards prohibit an individual from serving simultaneously on the Boards of Trustees of two chiropractic programs. Bob is not violating that standard. He serves as a member of the Board of Trustees at Logan Chiropractic College and as a member of the Board of Trustees at the University of Bridgeport, an academic institution which has among its various course offerings a chiropractic program. When I pointed that out to him, Arnold said he thought it was the same thing. When I told him he was mistaken, he was angry. I guess he presented the argument to gain a sense of my position.

(*The one thing I learned about academia, individuals play by the rules. If the standards read an individual is prohibited from serving on two Boards of Trustees of chiropractic programs simultaneously, that is the rule applicable to Board membership. If the standard prohibits simultaneous board member-*

ship on more than one governing board at a time, Dr. Matrisciano would be in violation of that standard. Based upon my reading of the CCE standards, there was no violation by UBCC.)

Bob is the only member of the Advisory Council to individually raise money and he is the person Bud and Arnold want to eliminate. Now that we are licensed, I wonder how long it will take for them to get rid of me.

I have learned one thing in the last 15 months. These guys talk about loyalty more than they live it.

(*Money was still the issue. Although Dr. Greenwood had agreed to underwrite the chiropractic program to the Board of Governors, the university did not have the money. The program had gotten licensed on the basis of a guarantee that could not be supported. If money was not forthcoming, the future credibility of the university with the Board of Governors would be destroyed. The ability of the college to hire personnel, order equipment and supplies, and function normally would not happen without an infusion of money.*)

1/21–I spoke with Bob who has his first Trustees meeting tomorrow. I hope he impresses the other board members and gets them to support us with money. I told him if Mollie Donavan donates some money, she should be put on the Advisory Council. He indicated she wouldn't want that. I said to put John Donavan (Mollie's son) on the board. Anything to get money. I asked if he had heard from Arnold. The answer was a predictable no. I wished him luck and told him I would speak to him tomorrow.

1/23–Met with Bart Block about the first trimester embryology and physiology courses. I also met with Jean Southard who assigned us an account number for tuition and application fees. I also deposited $375 in the account from five applications.

(*The January 25, 1991, program update report apprised the Advisory Council of the meetings which had been conducted to ensure the smooth transition of the College of Chiropractic into the functioning of the university. Over 200 applications had already been mailed to prospective students. Seven students had applied to the program and an additional 60 had submitted transcripts for review. Dr. Zolli reminded the members a library plan had to be submitted to the state by April 1.*)[2]

1/25–I met with Mike Bisciglia who wanted to know what was happening with fundraising. When I told him the dismal record, he advised me as to how the university conducts fundraising. He also indicated that Bud had told him these were some of the tactics that would be used to raise money for the College of Chiropractic. Mike suggested the committee hire a fundraiser to be assigned to Mike's staff whose sole purpose would be to raise money for the chiropractic program, at which point I shared with Mike the obvious, which I suppose somehow he had missed. The Chiropractic College Committee does not have the resources to pay me, where are they going to get the money to hire a fundraiser? I went on to say I was just about ready to throw in the towel. Mike said if I quit, there would be no school. I reiterated it doesn't look like there is going to be a school, anyway.

Mike said he would discuss the situation with Janet. About an hour later I received a call from Joan, in the president's office, telling me it was imperative the president meet with the Chiropractic College Committee, Carmen Tortora and myself on Monday. I knew this was not going to happen so I tried to talk Joan into arranging a conference call. After checking with the president, she agreed to a 12:00 p.m. conference call.

I called Marc Peyser who asked the call be moved to 1:00 p.m. Actually, he went on, the call would be better on Tuesday, before 1:00 or after 4:00, or anytime on Thursday. I called Bob Matrisciano who indicated a noon conference call would work, as long as it did not last for more than an hour. I then called Arnold. Marie, his receptionist indicated that he would be traveling to Dallas on Tuesday morning and he was busy all day Monday. I never spoke with Arnold. I realized there was not going to be a meeting.

The Advisory Council members wanted a Tuesday or Thursday meeting, and since I was now practicing on Tuesdays and Thursdays, and I would not be altering my schedule, this meeting would not happen.

I called Bob back and suggested he speak directly with Janet Greenwood and tell her our frustration. Furthermore, advise her that you (Bob) have identified people who are willing to contribute money, provided they be placed on the Advisory Council. Plain and simple, Arnold, Bud and Marc do not know money people, have no access to money people and to date have been woefully deficient in securing funding for this project. Not only have they not raised any money, they are a barrier to Bob getting money. Arnold objected to the people from whom Bob could get money because of their reputations. As a result, he did not want them associated with the college (or himself). If they wanted to control the membership of the Advisory Council they should have raised enough money themselves to ensure the programs stability and their control. Since they did not, other options must be explored. At this point in time, the school belongs to whomever puts up the money to make it happen.

I processed two more applications today. I spoke with Drs. Jeddeo Paul and Raymond Rappaport about the biochemistry courses. I wrote a letter to the Education Committee of the state legislature supporting chiropractors performing sports physicals. I also made appointments for next week.

I will not be here on Monday. I will be meeting with Larry O'Connell about our brochures and also because I cannot afford to drive up to Connecticut three times per week. At this point in time, I am owed $13,000 in back pay. If I am unable to recover a significant part of this money soon, I am in deep financial trouble. My resources are almost completely depleted and the expenses of opening my office are soon due.

On a positive note, my nephew Stephen and niece Kate Lynn were born today. Twins—the miracle of life in stereo. May they lead healthy, happy productive lives.

1/26–Arnold called to ask what I had arranged regarding the meeting with President Greenwood. He specifically wanted to know the status of Marc Peyser in regard to the meeting. I think Arnold senses that Bob is taking matters into his own hands and he is losing control. He then went on to ramble about the money from Fuji and if I knew the status and how he didn't know money people. I reminded him fundraising was not part of my job. I also stated that my job had been done and achieved the desired results. Fundraising had not been acceptable. He reiterated, if I wasn't going to be paid, I should not travel to UB and spend time there. Time? What about all the time I have spent on the program when not at UB? Not going to UB now, does not compensate me for the time and effort I have already expended. Arnold went on to say if this program takes off, I will be the dean. Being named dean of this program at this time is equal to being named captain of the *Titanic*.

I called Bob to tell him he might be getting a call from Arnold. While on the phone I advised him to make whatever arrangements necessary to secure funding for the program. Janet is unfamiliar with personalities within the chiropractic profession. Her allegiance is not to Bud, Marc or Arnold, her allegiance is to the College of Chiropractic and whoever can make that happen. President Greenwood will support whoever can come up with the money.

1/30– Mike Beecher (*VP of Finance*) let me into the building this morning and asked to meet with me. He wanted to know about fundraising. He expressed extreme disappointment and frustration in the Advisory Council's inability to raise funds and he further stated that perhaps the membership of the council should change. I expressed equal frustration and Mike stated the university would run the program whoever came up with the money. He is concerned I am looking to leave the program, which would be a major embarrassment to the university. I assured him that although I am angry, frustrated, disappointed and distressed, I would never abandon the program at this late date.

I then met with a prospective student. Then it was off to a meeting with the registrar. We discussed several issues of importance with regard to the functioning of the program. One item was grading. The university grades on a system of letter grades, pluses and minuses. Barbara (Gabianelli) will look into the possibility of the chiropractic program having its own grading system.

I can't describe the feelings I have when I speak with prospective students or university personnel. I try to project a positive attitude about the future of the program. At the same time, how can I lie to people about their future careers? So many people are basing their futures on the success of the program, yet there is no future for the program. I mean there is a future for the program, but it is tenuous at best. My intention has always been to establish a sound academic program. People cannot base their lives on my intentions. Are my intentions enough to nullify reality and permit me to lie? What about my colleagues on the Advisory Board? They have not worked to make this program successful, yet they are hanging on to control the enterprise when it becomes successful. They do not deserve to be part of this program in the future.

I met with a local chiropractor who would like to teach in the program. I spoke with another Connecticut D.C. who has been communicating with me for months and made arrangements with him to meet next Wednesday when I will explain the current status and arrange some kind of work schedule.

(After this doctor met with me and heard the status of the program, and the possibility of not being paid with any regularity, he withdrew his application for employment. I never saw or spoke to this individual again.)

I called Carmen Tortora to ask where he is on fundraising. He told me he would be able to tell me after Friday. I then called Bob to apprise him of the fundraising situation. Bob told me some of the individuals with whom he is speaking will not donate money as long as Arnold Cianciulli is involved with the Advisory Board. Alex Pireno in particular, a longtime friend of Bob's is willing to give him a $15,000 donation as soon as he is assured Arnold is not part of the program. Bob has attempted to reason with Alex, but for Alex, this is an emotional issue and reason will not prevail.

2/1–Provided Alex Pireno with a list of individuals from whom he wants to solicit funds. Both Bob and I think it is a bad move and told Alex the same, but he wants to do it anyway. The reason it is a bad move is these individuals have already been contacted and indicated they would not donate.

Received a call from Ed Coogan, D.C., who volunteered to help me at the university one day per week.

I spent the balance of the day answering correspondence and the phone. I met with Ted Schrager of the computer center and gave him a list of our needs.

When I got home I received a call from Bob. He told me NYSCA had printed a story in their newsletter that our program had failed and the university is bankrupt. These guys never stop.

(The February 20, 1991, program update requested the Advisory Council membership meet with President Greenwood, Mr. Tortora and myself at Waldemere Hall, her residence to discuss fundraising in addition to other topics. This was the last update to be mailed to Drs. Matrisciano, Cianci-

ulli and Peyser. The number of applications for admission had doubled and interviews were scheduled for prospective students. The only outstanding issue continued to be money.)[3]

Four hundred eighty-two applications had been mailed to prospective students in 24 states and Canada. Chiropractic education had come a long way from the days when schools were populated by students from the surrounding area. UBCC was reaching out across the country.

The deadline for the submission of the library plan was fast approaching and although work on the project had been ongoing, the report would not be released until payment in full was made for the work.

A decision had to be made regarding the membership of the Advisory Council. Dr. Matrisciano could ensure an influx of money into the program by inviting Alessandro Pireno, D.C. to be a member. Dr. Pireno would then invite other members to join, based upon their willingness to donate $15,000 to the college. When the dust cleared, the membership of the University of Bridgeport–College of Chiropractic Advisory Council consisted of:

Robert Matrisciano, D.C.,Chair   Alessandro Pireno, D.C.
John Shannon, Jr., D.C.   Mario Introna, D.C.
Sheldon Sinnett, D.C.   Gerald Stephens, D.C.
Thomas DeBari, D.C.

Dr. Pireno and his associates had contributed $75,000 to the college. Dr. Matrisciano recruited Sheldon Sinnett D.C. to the Advisory Council. The college had received $90,000 in approximately one month, which was more than it had received in the previous 14 months of fundraising. Bills were paid and the college was able to meet its financial commitments. However, the composition of the Advisory Council was problematic to local chiropractors. There were no Doctors of Chiropractic on the Council from the state of Connecticut. To solve this conundrum, a seat was created for the president of the Connecticut Chiropractic Association.

The Dean's Advisory Council consisted of former faculty from the Columbia Institute of Chiropractic: Robert Matrisciano, Alessandro Pireno, Mario Introna and Sheldon Sinnett. There is little doubt each of these men, in one way or another, were influenced by Ernest G. Napolitano. In addition, Gerald Stephens, D.C., who had actively participated in the Trustees struggle at the New York Chiropractic College donated the requisite funds to be named to the council. The connection between chiropractic's educational past and its future was well established in the composition of The University of Bridgeport–College of Chiropractic Dean's Advisory Committee. Would this group of individuals be able to embrace the future, and leave the past behind?

The first representative of The Connecticut Chiropractic Association on the Dean's Advisory Council was Richard Coopersmith, D.C. Dr. Coopersmith was an alumnus of the National College of Chiropractic and advised me he could not work against his alma mater. I tried to explain the UB program was not a threat to National, but my efforts with Dr. Coopersmith were to no avail. His participation on the council was reluctant and limited, but the seat had been established for participation by future representatives of the CCA.

The perception that one chiropractic program was a threat to another chiropractic program was a vestigial remnant of when chiropractic schools were proprietary. Because chiropractic schools are tuition dependent and supporting resources are limited, this sense of competition between schools continues.

While the influx of money staved off the imminent demise of the College of Chiropractic, it did not prepare the students, faculty and staff for the roller coaster ride they would endure until the graduation of the first class, due to the college being part of the University of Bridgeport.

(*The Bridgeport Post published a feature article in August 1991 announcing the opening of the chiropractic program. The projected goal for students was 60. The actual number of students who were accepted into the initial class was 20. There were 13 men and seven women in the class, all of whom possessed at least three undergraduate years of study. Sixteen possessed a baccalaureate degree. Of the 20 students accepted, 16 matriculated into the program at that time. Of the 16 students who started the program in September 1991, all graduated from the University of Bridgeport–College of Chiropractic. Ten were members of the inaugural graduating class. The others graduated in subsequent classes after having withdrawn from the program for one reason or another.*

Edwin Eigel, Jr. the provost of the university assumed the position of acting president in the fall of 1991, after Janet Greenwood, who championed the establishment of the College of Chiropractic at the University of Bridgeport resigned.)

After years of fiscal mismanagement, the University of Bridgeport was financially broke. As a result, the University Board of Trustees passed the following resolution:

"Resolved: The University will consider all responsible proposals including, but not limited to, more intensive fundraising, assistance from city, state and federal governments, affiliating with other accredited institutions of higher learning and discussions with the Professors World Peace Academy.

All of these shall be explored consistent with the University's educational mission and in a manner which will maintain the University's independence and the academic freedom of the faculty."[4]

Due to the dire circumstances faced by the university, administrators voluntarily accepted a 20% reduction in salary through the fiscal year ending June 30, 1992.[5] If the university was unable to raise several million dollars, or move to a less expensive location or restructure its debt, it would be forced to close within a year. The university administration was actively negotiating with Sacred Heart University and the University of New Haven for some type of affiliation. There was a proposal to turn the university over to the state, which was rejected by the state. There was a proposal for employee ownership of the university. There was a proposal to move Housatonic Community College (HCC) to the UB campus as a way of reducing expenses for UB and eliminating the need to build new facilities for HCC. All such proposals failed.

The University Board of Trustees unanimously rejected the offer by the Professors World Peace Academy in October 1991, responding to weeks of vocal opposition by students, faculty and alumni. *The Scribe*, the UB student newspaper, ran a front page article, the headlines of which read, "MOON U.? Reverend Sun Myung Moon convicted of tax evasion in 1984; Rev. marries 3,000 strangers at Madison Square Garden in 1988; Moon asks for UB's hand in marriage in 1991." Editorials and articles appeared in the *Bridgeport Post, Hartford Courant,* and local town publications. Several articles about the proposed affiliation were also published in the *Chronicle of Higher Education*.

During the course of these negotiations the UB Law School made arrangements to move and relocated to Quinnipiac University. The accreditation of the law school had been threatened because of the fiscal instability of the university. Once the possibility of affiliation with the Professors World Peace Academy (PWPA) became real, the dean of the law school, a vocal opponent of the affiliation, made the necessary arrangements and left UB. The director and faculty of the human nutrition program took up residence at the University of New Haven (UNH), as did two other senior faculty members who taught in the Dental Hygiene and Education Internship programs. Viable programs were pirated from the university without compensation. It looked as though UB was falling apart at the seams. The University of Bridgeport was never compensated in any way by the institutions which inherited these programs. It appeared that hostile takeovers occur in education the same way they do in business.

The crux of the matter was the fact that the PWPA was funded by the Unification Church, an organization which had a controversial history. The proposal offered by the PWPA was the infusion of money ($50,000,000) over a period of five years in exchange for appointing a majority of the members of the Board of Trustees.

(The University of Bridgeport was placed on probation by the New England Association of Schools and Colleges in December 1991.)

(The first program update sent to the new Advisory Council was dated March 6, 1992. In it, I attempted to inform the membership of what had been happening at UB. I was also able to inform them that all the students and faculty wanted the program to remain open. I didn't think it was prudent to tell them they had each contributed $15,000 to a school which was about to close.)[6]

The commitment and dedication of the students and faculty of the College of Chiropractic was inspiring and compelling. The petition committed the undersigned to attend the summer trimester and stated,

"We fully recognize that the opportunity for future trimesters beyond this summer is not assured. However we also understand that during this time, a concerted effort will be conducted to solidify the college's future."[7]

In April 1992, I formally requested a release be granted by the University of Bridgeport–Board of Trustees to allow the College of Chiropractic to negotiate independently with an institution willing to consider adding the College of Chiropractic to their university.[8] I had contacted several Connecticut institutions willing to discuss the possibility, however they wanted assurance they would not be sued by UB for "stealing" a program. The move of the senior faculty members to UNH had been controversial and had raised sensitivities in the academic world about pirating programs from weak institutions. My request was denied.

At the end of the spring semester a talent show was scheduled to help close out the semester on an upbeat note. One of the scheduled performers was the provost of the University, Lance Blackshaw, an excellent and accomplished pianist. On the day of the performance I had a meeting with Dr. Blackshaw and he asked if I would be attending the show that evening.

"I plan on attending but I don't know if I'll stay for the entire show. Driving round trip to Oyster Bay every day is wearing me out."

"But you have to stay until the end!"

"Would it mean that much to you?"

"Yes it would, ad to you too."

"Lance, I'll stay to the end of the show."

That night I attended the show. I slipped into a cushioned seat in the back of the Merten's theater and prayed I would be able to stay awake throughout the show. The show was excellent and everyone performing exhibited ability and enthusiasm for their art. Finally Provost Blackshaw sat at the piano and regaled the audience with several songs – played to perfection. He announced his final number would be of significance to some members of the audience and immediately went into "Please Release Me" a song popularized by Englebert Humperdinck. Those of us administrators in the audience got a laugh out of Dr. Blackshaw's performance and it was truly appreciated.

In the summer of 1992, the University of Bridgeport, with no other viable options available, completed negotiations with the Professors World Peace Academy. The financial crisis that had plagued the university for over a year appeared to be at an end. The college administration and faculty were focused on delivering the academic program while simultaneously preparing for accreditation by the state of Connecticut and the Council on Chiropractic Education.

While the agreement with the Professors World Peace Academy ensured the fiscal stability of the university and enabled it to remain open, it was nonetheless controversial. The nature of the controversy caused a reduction in the number of students attending the university as well as resignations by members of the faculty and staff. The money from the PWPA was coming into the university on a regular basis, but accounts payable was so far behind in their payments to vendors that some services and supplies were discontinued pending payment of outstanding invoices. Replacing vendors was difficult because the financial status of the university had been front page news in the publications throughout Connecticut. Venders were not willing to provide goods and services to the university for the privilege of being placed on a list which determined when they might be paid.

The state accreditation of the university was now in question. A group named The Coalition of Concerned Citizens (CCC), formed. This vocal, highly visible group opposed the agreement between UB and the PWPA. The group questioned the amount of academic freedom which would prevail on the UB campus and feared the possible indoctrination of UB students into the Unification Church. This controversy, like the financial crisis, was again played out in the media. For days, the university was the center of attention for advice by individuals or groups who were either in favor or opposed to UB being recertified for accreditation by the state. This advice was conveyed in editorials and special columns in the Bridgeport Post and other local publications.

In addition to conducting the academic program in an environment riddled with stress and instability, there were academic and regulatory issues with which to contend. The University of Bridgeport –College of Chiropractic had been licensed by the state, which qualified the program to accept students and conduct classes. Next, the state would have to accredit the program. State accreditation enabled the program to grant the Doctor of Chiropractic degree at the successful conclusion of the student's course of study. State accreditation was also a requirement for professional accreditation. Until UBCC was granted state accreditation, the eligibility documents required for starting the professional accreditation process could not be filed.

Work on state and professional accreditation occurred simultaneously. In addition, other issues needed to be addressed. Some states reserved the right to qualify graduates of a program to sit for licensure. As a result, this required UBCC to submit a separate report addressing the specific regulations of the state and hosting a state site team visit. New Jersey was one such state. There were four students in the inaugural class from New Jersey who wanted to return home to practice. In addition, New Jersey was the source of a large percentage of student inquiries. Approval by the state of New Jersey was critical for the success of the program.[9]

UBCC students had to become qualified to be eligible to sit for the National Board examinations. At the end of the first trimester of operations, I instructed Alan Hecht, D.C., who had been hired as Associate Dean, to contact the National Board of Chiropractic Examiners (NBCE) to ascertain the policies and procedures which would enable our students to take the boards. The response to our inquiry was highly motivating. The University of Bridgeport –College of Chiropractic had to secure state and professional accreditation, in addition to proving UBCC students were eligible to sit for licensure in one or more states.[10] The state of New Hampshire was the first state to accept UBCC students to sit for licensure. This approval was followed by Arizona.[11] The requirement "graduates are accepted for licensure in one or more states in the United States," had been met by UBCC.

These challenges paled in comparison to wondering if each day on campus would be the last for everyone involved in the college. Between the financial challenges of the university and the accreditation status of the university, there was a need for constant communication between the administration and the students.

Anthony Onorato, D.C., finally decided to leave NYCC. He joined UBCC as the Associate Dean in June 1992. His background as a seasoned administrator who left an established, accredited school to come to UBCC bolstered the confidence of the students and faculty. However, his confidence was shaken when I had to tell him he might not be getting paid his first paycheck because the university didn't have the money for payroll. He continued to work and never wavered in his commitment to the program.

My position as dean was filled with addressing the issues of: state and professional accreditation, state licensure eligibility, National Board eligibility and calming and communicating with the student body. There was also the matter of "proving" to the UB administration and faculty that a chiropractic program belonged in the university. To a degree I had made some progress in this area. When the director of the human nutrition program left UB and took the program and faculty to UNH, the UB administration asked me to administer the program until a permanent director could be found.

The number of meetings held at the university were staggering. Each meeting, no matter the agenda, usually focused upon the financial crisis and the latest rumors about the university's imminent demise. One day, at a meeting of the academic Deans and Directors with the provost, Bruce Skinner, the Dean of the Engineering School handed me a note with a napkin attached. The note stated, "This document was in my budget notes and may have historical value at UB." On the attached napkin was printed,

"The only difference between this place and the *Titanic* is they had a band."

I found this statement hysterical and passed it around the table to my colleagues. It appeared by their reactions that everyone thought the statement both hysterical and true. It was humor that could only be appreciated by people experiencing the same sense of impending doom.[12]

At the time of all this unrest, UBCC was conducting classes on a trimester system. Classes were in session year-round with little time off. Students were continually getting information from me as well as students from other programs about the dire situation faced by UBCC. For some reason, other chiropractic programs were acutely aware of what was happening in Connecticut to a new, non-accredited chiropractic program.

The stress of functioning in an environment with the resolution so many issues unclear reached its breaking point in November 1992. The inaugural class of the college was now in their fourth trimester, and they were anxious to sit for the National Boards. I met with the students to explain their status with regard to the NBCE tests as well as the accreditation process with the CCE. I explained the college was in the process of submitting documentation in support of our application for state accreditation. The college was in the process of communicating with various state chiropractic licensing boards seeking approval for UBCC graduates to sit for licensure.

For the first time, the students expressed disbelief in my explanations. The meeting was followed by a memo to each member of the class wherein I described the actions taken to allay their concerns.[13] I invited the Chairman of the Commission on Accreditation to the school to meet with the students. I indicated I would introduce the chairman, then leave the room. No member of the administration or faculty would be present during the presentation so as not to inhibit an open exchange between the students and the chairman.

Furthermore, I shared the information I had received from the Executive Director of the National Boards. Because there were subjects on Part I of the Boards UBCC students would not have sufficiently covered in the curriculum, they were ineligible to sit for the Boards until September 1993.

The November 1992 program update sent to the members of the Advisory Council stated, "Dr. Marino Passero, the Chair of the Commission on Accreditation of the Council on Chiropractic Education, addressed the student body. The purpose of his presentation was to explain the accreditation process and calm their fears about what they were reading and hearing daily about the financial posture of the University of Bridgeport."[14]

(*Not only were accreditation and National Boards on the minds of students, but basic necessities such as food and rent were issues also. The university was unable to process loans due to a procedural error that had been identified in a federal audit. During the investigation, the university deferred tuition payments but was unable to refund the balances due students.[15] The loan balance was the money calculated into the requested loan upon which students paid their regular living expenses. Students had become aware of this problem at the start of the fall term. Each time they went to the financial aid office they were told the problem was being reviewed and would be rectified shortly. After three months without resolution, the matter was reaching the critical point and was brought to my attention. I requested donations from the Advisory Council which would be placed in a restricted account to be used as loans for chiropractic students. Drs. Matrisciano and Sinnett provided funds for the Emergency Student Loan Fund and helped the college avert another catastrophe. Their generosity enabled the students to pay their living expenses. The money placed in the Emergency Loan Fund was repaid when the students received their refunds. Neither doctor accepted repayment but instead donated the money to the college, in case it was needed again.)*

President Edwin Eigel, Jr. received a letter from the Commissioner of the Department of Higher Education of the state of Connecticut dated April 27, 1993, wherein he was formally advised the College of Chiropractic had received state accreditation. State accreditation was contingent upon the program securing professional accreditation.[16]

(The New England Association of Schools and Colleges (NEASC), the regional accrediting agency of the University of Bridgeport, reported in its status statement on the University of Bridgeport dated March 10, 1993, "The Commission remains concerned that UB has not yet taken sufficient steps to develop and implement the necessary plans to fully address the many challenges it confronts in rebuilding the institution after years of declining resources leading to near financial collapse at the conclusion of the Spring 1992 semester. Among the variety of problems the university continues to face are substantial deferred maintenance, student recruitment and retention, the need to configure academic programs and related resources in light of institutional purposes and student demand, public relations, and finance including fundraising… . [T]he Commission believes the probationary status for the institution remains justified.")[17]

Work had been ongoing in the accreditation process. The information required by the state was the same as that required by the Council on Chiropractic Education. Since the Board of Governors had acted on UBCC's application approximately two weeks before the official notification letter was received by the university, the only piece of information needed to submit the college's eligibility document was a copy of Commissioner DeRocco's official letter. The college was officially notified by the Commission on Accreditation of the Council on Chiropractic Education that the college's eligibility document had been accepted in April 1993.[18]

A letter was sent to the president of the Association of Chiropractic Colleges (ACC), Gerard Clum, D.C. The purpose of the letter was to initiate a dialogue leading to the college being invited to join the organization. In the letter the status of the university, accredited but on probation, and the College of Chiropractic, accredited by the state of Connecticut, was explained. Also mentioned was the acceptance of the college's eligibility document by the CCE.[19]

Dr. Clum responded in a letter informing UBCC that at the March 30 meeting of the ACC the likelihood of the University of Bridgeport –College of Chiropractic seeking accreditation from the CCE had been discussed. The association bylaws were reviewed and consensus was reached that upon acceptance of the institution's eligibility document the institution would be eligible for ACC membership. In that letter, the University of Bridgeport– College of Chiropractic was welcomed into the Association of Chiropractic Colleges. The letter went on to say UBCC students were now eligible to participate in the ChiroLoan program for Title IV, Heal and ChiroLoan borrowing.[20]

For the first time other chiropractic programs were willing to accept the University of Bridgeport–College of Chiropractic as a sister institution. Until now, the college had been a curiosity discussed by representatives of the other schools. The college had been a possible source of transfer students when the university went out of business. The college was unlike any other chiropractic school, it was part of a university. It should be treated differently because of what it was. It should be treated differently until it was like all the other member institutions of the ACC.

Annual dues paid by member institutions was based on an amount per capita. The cost of annual membership dues for the UB College of Chiropractic was $146.66. A check request was filled out and the dues check was mailed. Several weeks later, the check was returned.[21] I called Dr. Clum and asked why the check had been returned and he explained the ACC Board of Directors had re-thought their decision to accept the membership of UBCC. According to the Board of Directors, the presidents of the other chiropractic colleges, membership in the ACC was based upon a program being accredited by the Council on Chiropractic Education. Dr. Clum had graciously provided me with a copy of the organization's bylaws when he originally welcomed the college into the ACC. I pointed out the bylaws read a program needed to be recognized by the CCE to qualify for membership, not be accredited. The option of suing the ACC was available, but my experience with legal matters had taught me there are better ways to solve acrimonious issues. My disappointment and that of the faculty, staff and students was palpable. The college would have to wait to become a member of the ACC.

My problem with the decision of the ACC Board of Directors was their misinterpretation of the written bylaws. While this action postponed the college's membership in the ACC, the actions of the individuals who comprised the board had more serious implications. The Boards of Directors of the ACC and CCE were composed of the same people, the presidents of the accredited chiropractic programs in the United States. If these people could misinterpret the ACC bylaws and postpone membership in one organization, what could stop them from potentially changing the academic standards of the CCE and postpone the accreditation of UBCC. If this were to happen, students currently studying at UBCC would not graduate from an accredited program. This would affect their ability to obtain a license and be a public relations nightmare for the college. It would compromise the college's ability to recruit students and raise questions regarding the quality of the program.

After I met with the senior members of the basic science faculty of the university and had been instructed about the value of clinical versus academic credentials, I applied for and was accepted into the Educational Leadership program at UB. This was the only doctoral level program offered by the university at the time. When the Board of Directors of the ACC was changing their minds about the criteria for programmatic eligibility, I was enrolled in ED MG 804–Constitutional, Legal and Political Issues Confronting Educational Leaders. I worked out my frustration with the situation by researching the legality of the action taken by the ACC Board of Directors. The end result of my research was my doctoral dissertation, titled *Professional Trade Associations, Accreditation Standards and Anti-Trust Legislation: Implications for the Chiropractic Profession.*

A synopsis of my dissertation was distributed to the Board of Directors of the CCE at my initial meeting with that organization. The Board of Directors passed a resolution which charged the Executive Committee with the responsibility of reviewing the matter and taking appropriate action. A year later the topic was still being discussed. One letter I received at that time was from Reed Phillips, D.C., PhD, president of the Association of Chiropractic Colleges. In his letter Dr. Phillips accurately stated the rationale for my theory, "was apparently stimulated by the fact the University of Bridgeport– College of Chiropractic was not allowed to participate in ACC activities until it had obtained CCE accreditation."[22] This letter and the others I received explained the reasons for the composition of the Boards of Directors of the organizations, but completely missed the unintended consequences that resulted from their rationale. In January 1999 the Council on Chiropractic Education issued a press release announcing a major restructuring had been approved by the Board of Directors.[23] On July 11, 1994 Dr. Clum, the president of the Association of Chiropractic Colleges congratulated me, the faculty, and the College of Chiropractic on achieving accredited status with the Commission on Accreditation of the Council on Chiropractic Education. Dr. Clum reiterated that CCE accreditation is a prerequisite to membership in the ACC, and stated if membership is desired, I should correspond with Dr. Clum as soon as possible.[24]

A letter was sent and UBCC attended the next meeting of the Association of Chiropractic Colleges in Davenport, Iowa. This meeting coincided with the Chiropractic Centennial Celebration. To celebrate UBCC's membership on the ACC Board of Directors, Dr. Ken Padgett, the treasurer of the ACC, who was aware of the financial challenges confronting the university, announced in front of the Board of Directors UBCC was delinquent in paying its dues. He did not have the courtesy to explain that UBCC had submitted a check for dues which was returned by the Association. The matter was rectified shortly after I returned to campus. This error by Dr. Padgett was yet another example of the pettiness which existed at other institutions as they came to grips with how they would relate to UBCC.

Neil Stern, D.C., was hired as the college's CCE consultant to guide

UBCC through the challenges of professional accreditation. Dr. Stern was eminently qualified for the assignment having achieved accredited status for the New York Chiropractic College and Parker College of Chiropractic. He also had served as the Chairman of the Commission on Accreditation of The Council on Chiropractic Education and helped write the academic standards used in the accreditation process.

He was very helpful in editing the self-study (the document submitted to the CCE before the site team visit) but the university administration benefited from his expertise when he performed a mock site team visit in anticipation of the team visit. Everyone at the college was appropriately prepared and nervous, but the university staff believed they were ready for the CCE, having been through regional and specialized accreditation visits before. A half hour of sitting with Neil Stern, answering his questions and providing knowledge of exhibits to validate the accuracy of their statements, convinced each administrator, staff and faculty member, more practice was required if the visit was to be a success.

The biggest challenge facing UBCC was the difference in our program from other programs—we were part of a university. The university of which we were part was on probation from the regional accrediting agency, although state accreditation had been extended through 1995. Dr. Stern's advice, always tell the truth and emphasize the benefits of university affiliation every time you can throughout the visit. The site team visit was conducted March 21-24, 1994. The members of the site team were:

William Fuller, Ed.D., Chairperson
Thomas Bergman, D.C., (Clinical Experience)
Michael Pelczar Jr., Ph.D., (Basic Sciences)
Donna Novack, B.S, B.A., (Finance)
Marcia Sasso, D.C., (Field Practitioner)
William DuMonthier, D.C., (Clinical Science/Research)

Each member of the team had received six binders of information. They detailed a narrative totaling approximately 300 pages of explanations and descriptions supported by 60 exhibits containing over 100 documents. Dr. Stern had prepared the college very well for the visit.

Dr. John Walters from the State of Connecticut, Department of

Higher Education was an observer during the visit. He was the recipient of all the documentation that had been sent to the Commission on Accreditation as well as the site team. The UB College of Chiropractic was the first time a chiropractic program was licensed and accredited by the state of Connecticut. No staff member of DHE had any experience with chiropractic education. This was the first experience for a DHE staff member to observe a site team accreditation visit for the Council on Chiropractic Education. At the end of the visit, Dr. Walters shared with me his thoughts on the chiropractic accreditation process. He thought the self-study and supporting documentation accurately reflected the status of the program. He thought the team came to campus very prepared, having read the self-study. He noted team members did not only know the area of the self-study for which they were responsible, but the entire document. The team reviewed exhibits thoroughly and correlated the information accurately and concisely in a draft report that would be submitted to the college shortly. Dr. Walters was favorably impressed by the team and the process.

The same could be said for the UB administration. The president, provost and vice presidents were impressed with the knowledge of team members and the thoroughness with which they conducted their interviews. The one question each of them had was, "Do they evaluate all schools the way they evaluated us?"

Having served on half a dozen site teams myself, I was able to answer in total honesty, "Yes, they do."

Dr. William Fuller had chaired the site team for the state in August 1990. There was a dramatic difference in the program now that students were inhabiting the buildings and interacting with faculty on a daily basis. The integration of the program within the university was more evident. Dr. Fuller's comments on page two of the site team report validated Dr. Stern's plan when he wrote:

"The college is unique in that it is part of university which provides many of the services included in a self-contained institution." He then went on to list the many benefits enjoyed by UBCC as part of the university. He concluded by saying:

"An additional strength of the college is the infectious enthusiasm of the students, faculty, board members and administration of the college for the chiropractic program. Most persons interviewed believe that the college will be in a leadership position among the other colleges of the university."[25]

Dr. Stern's analysis of the team report was equally thorough. The report, including the introduction numbered 29 pages. Dr. Stern's analysis took issue with 15 different points written on those pages. His most critical observation was that the team used the wrong version of the Standards in evaluating the program. The team used the January 1994 standards. The accreditation process had been ongoing for UBCC since April of the previous year, therefore the Standards which should have been used were those from January 1993. The college had made significant progress in addressing areas of the 1993 standards. In terms of the 1994 standards, the progress made was not as significant. At the end of his report, he proceeded to explain, in detail, how best to prepare the college response. He ended his explanation by writing,

"Prepare your response as if your life depended on it. One way or another it does! Either CCE–COA will kill you, or I will."[26]

The challenges and pettiness exhibited by individuals external to the University of Bridgeport, in the chiropractic profession, were equaled by the mentality that continued to exist within the university, especially relating to space. Clinical operations were scheduled to be opened on the third floor of the chiropractic building in time for the CCE site team visit. This location had been selected because it served the college's needs and required a minimal amount of renovation. The one drawback to using the third floor was that the anatomy laboratory would need to be relocated. The University of Bridgeport had been given a federal grant of $4 million dollars to renovate the Dana Science Building. In typical UB fashion, the money was spent before the project was complete. Knowing the anatomy laboratory needed to be moved, and space was available in the Dana Building, I visited the building one afternoon with Tony Onorato. We weren't in the building 30 seconds when we realized the southern end of the ground floor would be perfect to use for the anatomy lab. With the additional space, two chiropractic technique rooms and a classroom could be created. Now all we had to do was convince the occupants of that space to allow us to use it.

Because that part of the building hadn't been renovated there were no people on the ground floor. I suggested Tony and I go up to the second floor and scout additional space. As soon as we walked onto the second floor our presence was detected. To ensure everyone knew we were in the building I located a large laboratory space and exclaimed in a loud, excited voice, "This is it! This is the perfect space we need for the anatomy lab!"

We returned to the College of Chiropractic and went to our respective offices. The phone rang and it was the president of the university, Dr. Eigel.

"Frank, I understand you've been visiting Dana. What are you doing?"

"The clinic is opening on the third floor of the chiro building. I need to move the anatomy lab location."

"I'm aware of your needs for the upcoming accreditation visit, but you've created quite a stir with the basic science faculty in Dana."

"Ed, this is important, I need that space."

"Frank, the science faculty have plans for the area on the second floor you identified as perfect for the anatomy lab."

"What are they going to use it for," I inquired. The basic science faculty had indicated they had plans for the use of space in this building for years and the only results they had accomplished had been stopping the space from being used by anyone other than them.

"Frank, the basic science faculty want to help you."

Always being reasonable, I said, "Fine, let them give me the space I want and need."

"Frank, be reasonable. They have plans for this space. Ask them for anything else."

"Anything?"

"Yes, anything else."

"I want the southern end of the ground floor." The other end of the phone was silent.

I thought we had been disconnected, before Dr. Eigel stated, "That's more space than you need."

I replied, "It is right now, but consider this, the college is growing, we will need additional space in the next couple of years. I have the money to spend on the renovations right now and I certainly do not want to insult the basic science faculty by not accepting their offer to help the College of Chiropractic."

Game, set, match to the College of Chiropractic. Dr. Napolitano would have been proud. These higher education Ph.D.'s had been out-maneuvered by a chiropractor. And for the record, in a rare display of collegiality, the basic science faculty of the university actually helped the College of Chiropractic.

As stated in the March 25, 1994, program update to the Advisory Council, "As a side note, the people within the university were more than impressed with the depth in which the CCE team investigated every aspect of the program. I think our efforts all along, coupled with the intensity of the site team, have changed the opinions of people who once questioned whether chiropractic education belonged within a university."[27]

The Commission on Accreditation of the Council on Chiropractic Education awarded the University of Bridgeport–College of Chiropractic accredited status at the June 1994 meeting.[28] The award of initial accreditation was for a period of three years. Subsequently, the accredited status of the college was re-affirmed in 1997, 2002 and 2010. Each time the college has been re-affirmed, it has been for longer periods of time. In 1997, accreditation was granted for five years, and in 2002 for eight years. In 2010, the college was again re-affirmed for a period of eight years, which is the longest amount of time for which a chiropractic program can be accredited.

The presidents of several chiropractic colleges wrote congratulatory letters, as did the executive director of the Connecticut Chiropractic Association and Keith Overland, D.C., the president of the New England Chiropractic Council.[29]

As the college was enjoying victory in the area of accreditation, simultaneously the specter of professional misconduct reared its ugly head. The Advisory Council had been assembled to replace the original members who had been unable to raise the funds necessary to sustain the program.

The original members of the Chiropractic College Committee, became the Dean's Advisory Council. The university administration had entered into a written agreement with the Dean's Advisory Council defining the relationship between the parties. The original membership of the Advisory Council had been replaced, with the exception of Dr. Matrisciano. The agreement which had been created was now the responsibility of the new Advisory Council.

The person who most wanted to become a member of the Advisory Council was Alessandro Pireno, D.C. Dr. Pireno was a successful New York City practitioner who had staunchly supported Dr. Matrisciano during NYSCA's legal battles with insurance carriers. Dr. Pireno believed his experience in the field and the legal arena prepared him to be a member of the Dean's Advisory Council. As a chiropractor, Dr. Pireno could have been helpful to the dean advising him on professional issues. Unfortunately, Dr. Pireno and his associates did not fully understand their roles at the college. Based upon their experience in chiropractic education, they believed their status to be equal to that of a member of the Board of Trustees. Plain and simple, these individuals had donated money to save the program, and saw no reason to share their "power" with any new members who would need to be added to the council. The college needed to grow and become a regional presence. An Advisory Council, consisting exclusively of chiropractors from New York, would not satisfy the needs of the college, in this regard.

When the CCE site team members were on campus, they had difficulty understanding the role of the Advisory Council. Since the CCE standards make reference to a Board of Trustees as the governing body of an institution, are members of the Advisory Council Trustees? No, one member of the Advisory Council is appointed to serve on the Board of Trustees. Does the Advisory Council set policy for the College of Chiropractic? No, institutional policy is determined by the Board of Trustees. Does the Advisory Council appoint the dean of the college? No, the dean is appointed by the president from a list of candidates selected by the Advisory Council.

Drs. Pireno, Introna, Matrsiciano and Sinnett taught at the Columbia Institute of Chiropractic when Ernest G. Napolitano was both the Chairman of the Board of Trustees and the President of the school. They witnessed the power he possessed to affect the school, students, faculty and the chiropractic profession. Unfortunately, no one was able to explain the role of the Advisory Council to the new members. In addition, over the years, the roles of the administration and Boards of trustees had changed. What these individuals saw and experienced with Dr. Napolitano's leadership at both CIC and NYCC was now a relic of what had been acceptable behavior.

Dr. Matrisciano, the member of the Advisory Council who had been appointed to the Board of Trustees, requested he be relieved of the responsibility of being chair of the Advisory Council. He requested Dr. Pireno be appointed chair and I concurred. Dr. Pireno's first project was to revise the Advisory Council guidelines. I attempted to explain these guidelines had been bilaterally agreed upon by members of the Chiropractic College Committee and the UB administration. Any proposed revisions would need to be approved by the UB administration. I reminded Dr. Pireno the guidelines had been revised and ratified in 1991 by the Advisory Council while Dr. Matrisciano was chair. These revisions were essentially edits of the original document, which eliminated the job description of the dean and focused on the purpose and function of the council. The revisions were reviewed and ratified by the Advisory Council, then reviewed by the university attorney and members of the administration. Both groups were satisfied with the results, and the guidelines remained in force. Dr. Pireno was not pleased with my explanation and considered my position obstructionist. As a result, he and his colleagues boycotted meetings I called and the Advisory Council became inactive. The council members continued to receive monthly program updates and correspondence, without responding.

Chairman Pireno finally called a meeting in New York City. Invitations to the dean or UB administration were not extended. Revisions to the guidelines, proposed by Dr. Pireno were allegedly reviewed and passed by the membership. The revisions made to the guidelines created a monarchy of the chair position, created an Executive Committee, and violated the bylaws of the university.

On the basis of having "approved" guidelines, Dr. Pireno requested official stationary for use by himself and his appointees to the Executive Committee. A memo sent by Dean Zolli to Dr. Pireno, copied to the members of the Advisory Council, conveyed the official status of the Dean's Advisory Council. Official stationery is restricted to use by individuals authorized to act on behalf of the college/university and no member of the Advisory Council has that authorization.

Next, Dr. Pireno's lack of education experience became apparent when he informed the administration of the college, he and members of the Advisory Council would be visiting the college and wanted to review all records pertaining to the college's application for accreditation by the CCE. At that meeting, all records pertaining to the college's application for accreditation to the CCE, not just the self-study, should be available for review. In addition, the members of the Advisory Council expected to review faculty and staff personnel files, as well as faculty teaching schedules.In the fax transmission which outlined the demands of the Advisory Council, Dr. Pireno agreed not to use official stationary until the matter was clarified bu the university Board of Trustees.

Based upon the contents of this fax transmission it became obvious Dr. Pireno thought he could influence the hiring of faculty and staff. This was the way Nappy ran the Columbia Institue of Chiropractic and that's how he intended to control UBCC.He was totally unfamiliar with the policies and procedures of the University of Bridgeport, as well as regional and professional accreditation standards, all of which comply with federal and state regulations.

The visit of Dr. Pireno and the other members of the Advisory Council was cancelled when I advised Dr. Pireno the review of documents would be restricted to the self-study. If he requested a review of any additional documents I would need the approval of the university attorney.

Dr. Pireno's response to my correspondence, in addition to cancelling his visit, was to inform the UB administration that I had misrepresented my credentials on my curriculum vitae.On the basis of this allegation, I was summoned to a meeting with the president and provost of the university. At the meeting, the allegations made by Dr. Pireno were disprovedby my producing documents which confirmed the veracity of the information on my CV. As a result, the matter was dismissed.

While this conflict was raging, the college sponsored a one-day seminar featuring Professor Pran Manga who had previously published the Manga Report, a research study validating the cost effectiveness and clinical effectiveness of chiropractic care. After his lecture, which was on

"Chiropractic's Future as a Primary Care Provider," a panel discussion would be conducted with the audience. The members of the panel scheduled to appear were: Marino Passero, Arnold Cianciulli and Frank Zolli. All proceeds from the event would benefit the Chiropractic Research Fund. This event infuriated Dr. Pireno who was learning that although he had been able to have Dr. Cianciulli removed from the Advisory Council, he was unable to erase his positions of authority within the profession.[31]

Relations between the Advisory Council and the Dean were rapidly deteriorating. The Advisory Council was in need of diversification and activity. It was decided re- appointments would be made, in addition to new appointments. Inactive members would be thanked for their service and replaced. On this basis the membership of the Advisory Council changed and grew over the next few years. Sheldon Sinnett, D.C., who had been recruited by Dr. Matrisciano to donate money to the college, and provided funds for the Emergency Loan Fund was nominated for reappointment. Drs. Introna and Shannon were not active members of the Advisory Council and were not re-nominated for membership. The inactivity of Advisory Council members became the primary rationale for non-reappointment. In an appeal letter written to President Eigel protesting my action, Dr. Introna stated, "I am additionally disturbed at the notion of the university permitting a situation to exist in which a dean is authorized to unilaterally appoint or dismiss members of a body upon which the dean is or would be dependent for a recommendation for his reappointment." Appointment of the dean was the responsibility of the president when a vacancy in that position occurred. The Advisory Council was not authorized to recommend reappointment of the dean. It was apparent Dr. Introna did not understand the guidelines he ratified and by which he functioned as a member of the Advisory Council.[32]

Terms of office for the Advisory Council were three years and expired annually. On the basis of nomination and term expiration, the membership of the Advisory Council would change. New members would be recommended by sitting members of the Advisory Council and nominated by the dean to the president for appointment. A prerequisite for membership was residence in the northeast and a desire to be actively involved in chiropractic education.

Dr. Pireno was asked to submit his resignation from the Advisory Council. He never submitted his resignation, nor did he participate in college activities for the balance of his term in office. He was not re-nominated for membership on the Advisory Council.

The next challenge faced by the college was securing approval by the state of New Jersey for UBCC graduates to be eligible to practice. There were several issues evident which complicated this process. The straight/mixer controversy, though not defined in New Jersey law, was fundamental to the problem. The unfamiliarity of State Board members with academic regulations and common sense complicated the matter.

Though initial contact had been made with the New Jersey State Board of Chiropractic Examiners in October 1991, a site team visit was not conducted until December 1993. The visit started off poorly. Dr. DeMarco of the New Jersey Board requested a copy of the college's self-study which had been prepared for the upcoming CCE site team visit. I asked Dr. DeMarco why he wanted the CCE self-study which addressed the academic Standards of the Council on Chiropractic Education when his purpose on campus was to evaluate UBCC's compliance with New Jersey regulations. Dr. DeMarco had been a strong, vocal supporter of straight chiropractic schools, and his philosophical preference was not consistent with the mission of the University of Bridgeport–College of Chiropractic. My refusal to provide Dr. DeMarco, and the other team members Harold Doe, D.C., and Priscilla Adams-Church, a copy of the CCE self-study, though not a violation of any regulations, set the tone for the visit.

The final report the team submitted listed seven recommendations to be implemented by UBCC. A copy of the team report was received by the college, along with a cover letter dated June 23, 1994. In the cover letter the college was notified "an on-site, follow-up, unannounced visit would be conducted sometime in late 1994."[33]

The first UBCC graduation was scheduled to be conducted in December 1994. If the next New Jersey site team visited campus in fall 1994, there was little chance a decision on eligibility for UBCC students would be made in time for the January 1995 licensing examination. The last visit was conducted in December 1993 and the college received a copy of the report six months later! The timing of the process was problematic, as was the content of the report. In an attempt to address the concerns of the New Jersey Board of Chiropractic Examiners and expedite the licensure eligibility of UBCC graduates a response was developed and submitted to the New Jersey Board.

In the response the board was notified that UBCC had been granted accreditation by the Commission on Accreditation of the Council on Chiropractic Education. The response further addressed each of the recommendations made in the state report. Although some of the recommendations were based on inaccuracies reported by the team members, they were addressed respectfully.[34]

After mailing the response to the New Jersey Board, I called Rick Rapone, one of the new appointees to the Dean's Advisory Council. Rick was a New Jersey attorney who had successfully worked with chiropractors for years. I asked him to obtain a temporary restraining order (TRO) against the New Jersey Board of Chiropractic Examiners prohibiting the January licensing examination from taking place until the eligibility of UBCC graduates was decided. The TRO was never obtained or necessary.

(The June 21, 1994, program update to the Advisory Council announced to the membership the college's accreditation by the CCE. The report acknowledged the contributions of individuals within the college who had distinguished themselves, in my opinion, during the accreditation process. Also acknowledged in the update were the faculty of the college, the staffs of the various support services offered by the university, the President and Vice Presidents, the Board of Trustees and the members of the Advisory Council. This program update was somewhat bittersweet. By the time it was sent, some of the members whose financial contributions had enabled the college to survive had already been replaced. Within two years the individuals who had contributed money and saved the college from extinction all had been replaced.)[35]

In anticipation of the college's first graduation, the establishment of the Ernest G. Napolitano Award was proposed to the university administration. The description of the award read:

Ernest G. Napolitano was a giant in the chiropractic field. A graduate of the Palmer College of Chiropractic, Dr. Napolitano led the Columbia Institute of Chiropractic from two small brownstones in Manhattan, to a

50-acre campus with modern facilities on Long Island. In the process he transformed the Columbia Institute of Chiropractic into the New York Chiropractic College.

During this time, Dr. Napolitano developed the reputation of being in service to the profession. He was deeply involved in all areas of chiropractic education and politics. In addition to being a statesman, he was an innovator.

One of his innovations was the human nutrition program started at the University of Bridgeport. Through the efforts of Dr. Napolitano, UB accepted the challenge of starting a Master's of Science Degree in Human Nutrition, which today is a major program at the university.

Eligibility for the award would be based upon evidence of significant contributions to the chiropractic profession and the University of Bridgeport.[36]

Of the 16 students who entered the University of Bridgeport–College of Chiropractic in the fall of 1991, ten participated in the commencement exercises which were conducted on December , 1994. The commencement speaker was Louis Sportelli, D.C. Dr. Neil Stern received an honorary degree from the University of Bridgeport in recognition of his tireless work in helping the college secure professional accreditation. Robert Matrisciano D.C. was the recipient of the first Ernest G. Napolitano Award. This award would be bestowed one more time, in 1999. The recipient was Marino Passero, D.C.

The inaugural graduating class of the University of Bridgeport – College of Chiropractic consisted of:

> Gina Carruci - Connecticut
> Ardee Frizzell Davis - New Jersey
> Todd Davis - Massachusetts
> Michael DiMauro - Massachusetts
> Stephen Fowler - Connecticut
> Michael Gaccione - New Jersey
> Karl Nixdorf - New Jersey
> Angela O'Hara - Connecticut
> Frederick Stinner - New Jersey
> Behjat Syed - Connecticut

There were four graduates from Connecticut and New Jersey, and two from Massachusetts. For all the attention UBCC received from NYCC, there were no graduates from the state of New York.

It took 98 years from the inception of chiropractic education in 1896, to the first commencement exercises of a chiropractic program conducted at a university in 1994. During that time span, chiropractic education had to overcome challenges faced by all academic institutions, and some unique to chiropractic. Improving the quality of facilities, faculty, the curriculum, the library and adding sufficient parking, are rites of passage experienced by all institutions of higher learning. Addressing these challenges in the ever-present shadow of medical oppression and adverse medical influence requires special qualities.

My efforts at starting a chiropractic program at the University of Bridgeport were based upon my experience as a chiropractor and administrator at the New York Chiropractic College. I accepted the position to correct a long standing injustice in higher education. The injustice was based upon ignorance and prejudice, but it persisted nonetheless. Little did I realize that human frailty in the form of jealousy would also play a part in the process.

The first challenge of the assignment was convincing the university faculty that a chiropractic program was worthy of university affiliation. The faculty were educated individuals highly influenced by medical propaganda. The same was true for the staff at the State of Connecticut Department of Higher Education. Hard work and substantive documentation to comply with licensure and accreditation criteria was sufficient to do the job.

The progress of the college was closely monitored by the other chiropractic schools. Some of the programs also actively worked to make the process more difficult. Perhaps the honor of establishing the first university based chiropractic degree program in the United States was supposed to go to an established school. Since UBCC was founded, eight of the existing chiropractic colleges which were single purpose, stand- alone institutions, morphed into becoming universities.

Utilizing technical knowledge and experience to overcome the obstacles of acceptance, licensure and accreditation, were essential but the challenges of funding for both the college and university required more than technical knowledge. Financial instability in the college plagued the project from its inception. The unraveling of the university's finances became apparent after the college had gained a foothold in the world of higher education.

The financial challenges needed to be overcome required tenacity, commitment, passion, and common sense. Each of these qualities, individually or in combination, exhibited by university and college personnel enabled chiropractic education to become part of higher education in the United States.

To achieve licensure and accreditation in higher education, specific criteria must be addressed. The criteria are listed in the licensure and accreditation applications provided by the state. To achieve professional accreditation specific criteria, outlined by the professional accrediting agency, must be addressed. To succeed in higher education a knowledge of criteria and procedure is mandatory. However, tenacity, commitment, passion and common sense, none of which is taught in the classroom, are essential components in achieving success. Because they are not taught in the curricula of formal education at any level, their use is not restricted to being applied specifically in the process of securing a place in higher education.

The journey of the Columbia Institute of Chiropractic to becoming the New York Chiropractic College required tenacity, commitment, passion and common sense. The growth of the New York Chiropractic College in securing an absolute state charter required tenacity, commitment, passion and common sense. The founding of the University of Bridgeport – College of Chiropractic required tenacity, commitment, passion and common sense. It appears the chiropractic profession maintained the requirements necessary to be part of higher education all along – the only thing lacking was the opportunity. That is no longer true.

Notes

The following section provides abbreviations which occur in the text, as well as footnotes which are numbered in the chapters. The footnotes listed in this section are identified by the chapter in which they are found.

AAOS – American Academy of Orthopedic Surgeons
AAPMR – American Academy of Physical Medicine and Rehabilitation
AAUP – American Association of University Professors
ACA – American Chiropractic Association
ACC – Association of Chiropractic Colleges
ACP – American College of Physicians
ACS – American College of Surgeons
AMA – American Medical Association
AOA – American Osteopathic Association
ASCI – Atlantic States Chiropractic Institute
BOG – Board of Governors, State of Connecticut, Department of Higher Education
CCA – Connecticut Chiropractic Association
CCC – Columbia College of Chiropractic (Chapter 1)
CCC – Concerned Citizens Coalition (Chapter 5)
CCCW – Cleveland Colle of Chiropractic – West
CCE – Council on Chiropractic Education
CIC – Columbia Institute of Chiropractic
CINY – Chiropractic Institute of New York
CMS – Chicago Medical Society
COA – Commission on Accreditation
DOH - Department of Higher Education
DHEW – Department of Health, Education and Welfare
ICA – International Chiropractors Association
IME – Independent Medical Examination
IMS – Illinois Medical Society
JCAH – Joint Commission on the Accreditation of Hospitals
LIE – Long Island Epressway
NEASC – New England Association of Schools and Colleges

NBCE – National Board of Chiropractic Examiners
NCC – National College of Chiropractic
NECC – New England Chiropractic Council
NYCC – New York Chiropractic College
NYIT – New York Institute of Technology
NYSCA – New York State Chiropractic Association
PCA – Pennsylvania Chiropractic Association
PCCW – Palmer College of Chiropractic – West
PSC – Palmer School of Chiropractic
PWPA – Professor's World Peace Academy
RCA – Recognized Candidate for Accreditation
SACS – Southern Association of Colleges and Schools
SGA– Student Government Association
SORSI – Sacro Occipital Research Society International
TRO – Temporary Restraining Order
UB – University of Bridgeport
UBCC – University of Bridgeport College of Chiropractic
USOE – United States Office of Education

Chapter One

1. *B.J. of Davenport: The Early Years of Chiropractic* p.14, Joseph C. Keating Jr., 1997, Davenport, Iowa, Association for the History of Chiropractic
2. ibid pgs.23-24
3. *Chiropractic: History and Evolution of a New Profession* p.60 Walter I. Wardwell, 1992, St. Louis, Missouri, Elsevier Mosby – Year Book Inc.
4. *Chiropractic: An Illustrated History* p. 341, Dennis Peterson, Glenda Wiese, 1995, St.Louis, Missouri, Elsevier Mosby Year Book, Inc.
5. ibid p.341
6. Ferguson,Alana, Wiese, Glenda 1988, How Many Chiropractic Schools, An Analysis of Institutions that Offered the D.C. Degree, *Chiropractic History 8(1), pgs. 26 - 36*
7. *Chiropractic: History and Evolution of a New Profession* p.168 Walter I.

Wardwell, 1992, St.Louis, Missouri,Elsevier Mosby – Year Book Inc.

8. ibid p.169

9. ibid p.163

10. *A History of Chiropractic Education in North America* p. 157, Joseph C. Keating Jr., Alana K. Callender, Carl Cleveland III, 1998, North Tazewell, Virginia, The Association for the History of Chiropractic, Council on Chiropractic Education

11. ibid p.158

12. ibid p.13

13. ibid p.159

14. ibid p.160

15. ibid p.163

16. *Chiropractic: An Illustrated History* p. 393, Dennis Peterson, Glenda Wiese, 1995, St.Louis, Missouri, Elsevier Mosby Year Book, Inc.

17. ibid p.393

18. Columbia Institute of Chiropractic Bulletin 1965 – 68 p.10

19. *Chiropractic: History and Evolution of a New Profession* p. 143 Walter I. Wardwell, 1992, St. Louis, Missouri, Elsevier Mosby – Year Book Inc.

20. 1954 Columbian – year book of the Columbia Institute of Chiropractic and the Columbia College of Chiropractic

21. *B.J. of Davenport: The Early Years of Chiropractic* p. 86, Joseph C. Keating, Jr.,1997, Davenport, Iowa, Association for the History of Chiropractic

22. *Chiropractic: An Illustrated History* pgs. 408 – 409, Dennis Peterson, Glenda Wiese, 1995, St. Louis, Missouri, Elsevier Mosby Year Book, Inc.

23. ibid p. 409

24. *A History of Chiropractic Education in North America* p. 162, Joseph C. Keating Jr., Alana K. Callender, Carl Cleveland III, 1998, North Tazewell, Virginia, The Association for the History of Chiropractic, Council on Chiropractic Education

25. *Chiropractic: An Illustrated History* p. 408, Dennis Peterson, Glenda Wiese, 1995, St. Louis, Missouri, Elsevier Mosby Year Book, Inc.

26. *Chiropractic: History and Evolution of a New Profession* p. 95 Walter I. Wardwell, 1992, St.Louis, Missouri, Elsevier Mosby – Year Book, Inc.

27. Columbia Institute of Chiropractic Bulletin 1962 – 64, p. 10

28. *Chiropractic: An Illustrated History* p. 187, Dennis Peterson, Glenda Wiese, 1995, St.Louis, Missouri, Elsevier Mosby Year Book, Inc.
29. *A History of Chiropractic Education in North America* p.144, Joseph C. Keating Jr., Alana K. Callender, Carl Cleveland III, 1998, North Tazewell, Virginia, The Association for the History of Chiropractic, Council on Chiropractic Education
30. Columbia Institute of Chiropractic Bulletin 1962 – 64, p.9
31. *A History of Chiropractic Education in North America* p. 129, Joseph C. Keating Jr., Alana K. Callender, Carl Cleveland III, 1998, North Tazewell, Virginia, The Association for the History of Chiropractic, The Council on Chiropractic Education
32. ibid p.162
33. 1968 Columbian – year book of the Columbia Institute of Chiropractic
34. Columbia Institute of Chiropractic Bulletin 1974 – 77 pgs. 6 – 9
35. Columbia Institute of Chiropractic Bulletin 1971 – 74 p. 5
36. Columbia Institute of Chiropractic Bulletin 1974 – 77 p. 5
37. Columbia Institute of Chiropractic Bulletin 1975 – 76 p. 9
38. Columbia Institute of Chiropractic Bulletin 1977 – 78 p. 9
39. New York Chiropractic College Bulletin 1978 – 80 p. 14
40. Napolitano Correspondence to Administrative Staff – Stern Catalogue Responsibilities 7/27/77
41. Napolitano Correspondence – Levittown Inspection 2/25/85
42. Napolitano Correspondence – Zolli Report 2/8/77
43. Napolitano Correspondence – Zolli SGA President 9/5/78
44. New York Chiropractic College Bulletin 1987 – 88 (Board of Regents Absolute Charter) p.23
45. Bundy Aid www.cicu.org
46. Napolitano Correspondence – Zolli 6/5/80
47. Napolitano Correspondence – Discontinuing Chief of Staff Position 6/5/80
48. Brief History of the New York Chiropractic College p.5
49. Ibid p. 6
50. *A History of Chiropractic Education in North America*, p.164, Joseph C. Keating, Jr., Alana K. Callender, Carl Cleveland III, 1998, North

Tazewell, Virginia, The Association for the History of Chiropractic, The Council on Chiropractic education.

51. Minimum Wage – www,dol.gov/whd/minwage/chart.htm
52. Napolitano Correspondence Zolli 4/18/85
53. Gibbons Correspondence Napolitano 4/15/85
54. New York Chiropractic College Bulletin 1987 - 88 (Middle States Accreditation) p. 23
55. Napolitano Correspondence Chair of Clinical Sciences 10/1/84
56. Napolitano Correspondence Zolli executive chair   2/14/85

Chapter Two

1. Columbia Institute of Chiropractic Bulletin 1962 – 64 p.7
2. Columbia Institute of Chiropractic Bulletin 1965 – 68 p.9
3. Columbia Institute of Chiropractic Bulletin 1962 – 64 p.7
4. Columbia Institute of Chiropractic Bulletin 1962 – 64 p.7
5. Incorporation Papers – Drs. Heuser & Pennell
6. Columbia Institue of Chiropractic Bulletin 1975 – 76 p.9
7. Dr. Pennell's letter to Dr. Napolitano – 7/26/80
8. Dr. Pennell's Nominating letter to the Board of Trustees -7/28/80
9. Theodore Roosevelt: Citizenship in a Republic, speech delivered 4/23/10 at Sorbonne in Paris, France
10. DeGiacomo letter to Langilotti – 4/7/86
11. Langilotti – Zolli letter exchange – 4/10/86
12. Dr. Stern Budget Letter to Board of Trustees – 11/18/85
13. Dr. Stern letter to Chairman Nystrom – Free Standing Institution – 11/17/86
14. Dr. Sullivan letter to Dr. Stern – 1/29/86
15. Dr. Sullivan letter to Chairman Forte – 2/4/86
16. Ibid p. 2
17. Dr. Napolitano letter to Dr. Heuser – 3/18/85
18. Dr. Napolitano letter to Mr. Zerdin – 3/29/85
19. Dr. Pennell letter to Dr. Napolitano – 7/26/80
20. Student Petition to NYCC Board of Trustees – 4/28/86
21. Petitions to New York State Education Department (Administration, Faculty, Alumni) 4/30/86

22. Deputy Commissioner Nolan letter to SGA president Montalbano – 5/14/8
23. Senator Johnson letter to Chancellor Barrell – 5/19/86
24. Dr. Matrisciano letter to NYSCA Membership – 6/2/86
25. Dr. Pennell letter to Clients – 6/3/86
26. NYCC Response to Pennell letter 6/8/86
27. Stern letter to Deputy Commissioner Nolan – 6/5/86
28. Zolli letter to Stern – 4/9/86
29. Regents' Committee Report p.3
30. Ibid p.4
31. Ibid p.8
32. Ibid p.9
33. Ibid p. 13
34. Ibid p.14 & 15
35. Ibid p. 16 & 17
36. Ibid p. 19
37. Ibid p. 19
38. Ibid p. 20
39. Ibid p.21
40. Wein Witness List
41. Regents' Committee Report p. 22
42. Ibid p. 24
43. Ibid p. 25
44. Ibid p. 25
45. Ibid p.29
46. Ibid p.29
47. Ibid p.29
48. Ibid p. 30
49. Ibid p.30
50. Sullivan letter to Stern – Removal of Probation – 1/29/87

Chapter Three

1. Stern letter to Nystrom – Trustee Blake 2/2/87
2. Stern letter to Lopez – Alumni 12/12/86

3. 1968 Columbian – Yearbook of the Columbia Institute of Chiropractice

4. Stern letter to Nystrom = NYIT Contract/Board Terms 10/14/86

5. Stern letter to Nystrom – Free -Standing Institution 11/17/86

6. Stern letter to Board – Initial Budget 11/18/885

7. Stern letter to Board – Line Item Explanation 12/15/86

8. The Case for Conflict of Interest – undated

9. *A History of Chiropractic Education in North America*, p.181 – Keating, Joseph Jr., Callendar, Alana, Cleveland, Carl III, 1998, North Tazwell, Virginia, The Association for the History of Chiropractic, The Council on Chiropractic Education

10. The Case for Conflict of Interest – undated

11. Steiner letter to Board – Nystrom 2/13/87

12. McAndrews Resignation Letter – 2/10/87

13. Ibid – 2/10/87

14. Nelson Report to the Board of Trustees – 2/14/87

15. Stern letter to Lopez – Alumni 12/12/86

16. NYCC Press release – 6/23/87

17. Ibid – 6/23/87

18. Wein Witness List

19. NYCC Press Release – 6/23/87

20. Stern letter to Pappas – Planning 6/9/87

21. *Chiropractic: History and Evolution of a New Profession*, p.168, Walter I. Wardwell – 1992, St. louis, Missouri, Elsevier Mosby – Yearbook Inc.

22. Stern letter to Lopez – Hinshaw 7/8/87

23. Stern letter to Sullivan and Cromwell – Policies/Procedures 11/6/86

24. Stern letter to Nystrom – Policies 6/9/87

25. History of Staff decisions at NYCC – 6/9/89

26. *A History of Chiropractic Education in North America*, p.181, Keating, Joseph C. Jr., Callndar, Alana, K., Cleveland, Carl III, North Tazewell, Virginia, The Association for the History of Chiropractic, The Council on Chiropractic Education 1998

27. History of Staff Decisions at NYCC – 6/9/89

28. Long Range Planning Minutes – 8/11/87

29. Ibid – 8/11/87
30. Ibid – 8/11/87
31. History of Staff Decisions at NYCC 6/9/89
32. Ibid – 6/9/89
33. NYCC Press Release – 6/23/87

Chapter Four

1. UB Press Release – 10/20/89
2. Eigel to Passero Memo – 8/16/89
3. January Program Update – 1/19/90
4. February Program Updates – 2/14 & 2/23/90
5. Genesis Fund Brochure Invoice – 4/3/90
6. Advisory Council Guidelines – 3/22/90
7. March Program Updates - 3/9 & 3/23/90
8. Medical School Admission Requirements 1990 – 91 pgs. 144 – 47; 174 – 75; 190 – 95; 262 – 63; One DuPont Circle NW, Washington, DC 41st edition
9. April Program Update – 4/16/90
10. Response to State Licensure Application – 5/30/90
11. May Program Updates - 5/9 & 5/25 90
12. June Program Updates – 6/13 & 6/15 & 6/22/90
13. July Program Updates – 7/6 & 7/23/90
14. Zolli letter to Feldman – 8/22/90
15. Greenwood letter to Padgett – 8/27/90
16. August Program Update – 8/30/90
17. September Program Updates – 9/17 & 9/20/ 90
18. October Program Updates – 10/1& 10/26/90
19. November Program Update – 11/6/90
20. President Greenwood lettr to Governor O'Neill – 9/26/90
21. December Program Update – 12/7/90

Chapter Five

1. Program Update – 1/7/91
2. Program Update – 1/25/91

3. Program Update – 2/20/91
4. UB Board of Trustees Resolution –Undated
5. Eigel Letter – Pay Reduction – 1/13/92
6. Program Update -3/6/92
7. Student Petition to Remain at UBCC – 3/3/92
8. Zolli Release Request Letter – 4/8/92
9. Zolli Letter to DeMarco – New Jersey Regulations – 10/9/91
10. NBCE Letter to UBCC – 12/13/91
11. State Licensure Eligibility Validation Letters – 6/9/93 & 6/22/93
12. Dean Skinner Note/Napkin – undated
13. Zolli Memo Addressing Student Concerns – 11/20/92
14. Program Update – 11/30/92
15. State of Connecticut Accreditation Resolution – 4/27/93
16. NEASC Status Report – 3/10/93
17. Commissioner DeRocco letter to President Eigel – 4/27/93
18. CCE Eligibility Confirmation Letter – 4/22/93
19. Zolli letter to Clum – 4/30/93
20. Clum Response to Zolli – 5/5/93
21. ACC Check Return Memo – 10/15/93
22. Phillips Letter – 12/2/96
23. CCE Restructuring Announcement – 1/29/99
24. Clum letter to Accredited UBCC
25. CCE Site Team Report – 3/21 – 24/94
26. Stern Analysis of Site Team Report – 3/31/94
27. Program Update – 3/25/94
28. CCE Accreditation Resolution – 8/23/94
29. Congratulatory Letters – 7/6/94 & 6/29/94 & 7/7/94
30. Pireno Request Letter – 4/14/94
31. Program Update – 4/21/94
32. Introna Letter – 6/20/94
33. New Jersey Cover Letter – 6/23/94
34. Response to New Jersey Report – 7/5/94
35. Program Update – 6/21/94
36. Napolitano Award – 8/26/94